THE CANCER PARENT'S HANDBOOK

the Cancer Parent's Handbook

What Your Oncologist Doesn't Have Time To Tell You

LAURA DEKRAKER LANG-REE

the publishing CIRCLE.

the publishing CIRCLE™

Send permission requests to the publisher at:
admin@thepublishingcircle.com.
Attention: Permissions Coordinator
Regarding Laura DeKraker Lang-Ree

DISCLAIMER: The Publisher and the Author make no representations or warranties with respect to the accuracy or completeness of the contents of this work and specifically disclaim all warranties, including, without limitations, warranties regarding fitness for a particular purpose. No warranty may be created or extended by sales or promotional materials. The advice and strategies contained herein may not be suitable for every situation. This work is sold with the understanding that the Publisher is not engaged in rendering medical, legal, accounting, or other professional services. If professional assistance is required, the services of a competent professional person should be sought. Neither the Publisher nor the Author shall be liable for damages arising here.

The fact that an organization or website is referred to in this work as a citation and/or a potential source of further information does not mean the Author or Publisher endorses the information the organization or website may provide or recommendations it may make. Further, readers should be aware that Internet websites listed in this work may have changed or disappeared between when this work was written and when it is read. The publisher is not responsible for the Author's website, other mentioned websites, or content of any website that is not owned by the Publisher.

The names of some individuals referenced in this book have been changed to protect and honor their privacy.

All content is the Author's opinion only.

Published by The Publishing Circle
www.thepublishingcircle.com

THE CANCER PARENT'S HANDBOOK: WHAT YOUR ONCOLOGIST
DOESN'T HAVE TIME TO TELL YOU
FIRST EDITION
ISBN   978-1-955018-66-1 (PAPERBACK)
ISBN   978-1-955018-96-8 (HARDCOVER)
ISBN   978-1-955018-71-5 (LARGE PRINT)
ISBN   978-1-955018-70-8 (eBOOK)

Stacey Teischer

BSN, RN, MSN, PNP, AOCNP, DNP, Oncology

"This book is a must-read for everyone who knows a child who had cancer or is starting their cancer journey. The Tips and Tools are incredibly valuable and not seen in any other literature or spoken to you by your oncology providers because they don't know what it is like to live with a child who has cancer. This book shares vital information on how to prevent long term side effects for the survivor, which is often overlooked until it is too late. I love how this book addresses the WHOLE family and provides suggestions on how to help everyone thrive during this incredibly difficult time. It is beautifully written and impossible to put down—you will be surprised how uplifted and empowered you will feel from this book."

Dr. Gary Dahl, MD

Pediatric Oncology & Hematology, Lucile Packard Children's Hospital at Stanford

Professor Emeritus, Stanford University Medicine

Architect, The Health After Treatment (HAT) Program at Lucile Packard

"I read the book and found that it will be incredibly necessary for all of our families to have their hands on. Learning how to just be there, as a parent, family, caregiver and healthcare provider is found in this book."

"Everyone needs help along the way. There's so many things you can learn that Laura has experienced. You'll get that in the Cancer Parent's Handbook. This will give you help. We could all use help. Reminders. I don't think I've ever seen anything like this in a book."

Pam Simon, MSN, CPNP, CPON

Nurse Practitioner & Program Manager SAYAC (Stanford Adolescent and Young Adult Cancer Program)

This book is full of soooo much valuable information written from a Mom with experience and passion! Childhood cancer treatment is complicated and this handbook is a tool to help guide parents through a very difficult time.

Jill Whisler, Cancer Mom of a 10-year-old.

"This Guide is amazing and easy to read! The bullet points of "how-to's" are packed with incredible gems that can be critical in getting you and your family through this journey."

Dedication

The Cancer Parent's Handbook is dedicated to all the families whose children will be diagnosed with cancer. I'm here for you. Your voices, your stories, and your children matter. You are warriors, one and all, and I'm so honored to be a part of your world during this life-changing experience. May this book bring you help, direction, inspiration, peace, and hope.

Acknowledgements

When our daughter was diagnosed with childhood leukemia in 1999, the lack of information for parents navigating everyday life with cancer was heartbreaking and utterly frustrating. Thanks to our support group, Jacob's Heart Cancer Supportive Services, and the bevy of amazing moms I met in Clinic D and online, I eventually found my way and my strength. But it should not have been so hard, and I was pissed off, sure that everything I needed to know about how to navigate life with cancer at home and the hospital was there, *somewhere*, for all cancer parents. But it wasn't and still isn't—until now.

During treatment, this frustration turned constructive, and before long, I knew I had a book in me. I saw it as my way of giving back—someday. That someday is now! I'm eternally grateful to the people who helped me keep this flame alive and encouraged me to bring it into reality during the quiet of COVID-19.

My ability to publish *The Cancer Parent's Handbook* combines my ambition and desire to help others with the uncanny destiny of meeting one person after another, links in a chain that ultimately connected me to getting this book into your hands. None of it felt like a coincidence, as each person along the way simply led me here in the most intentional and magical way.

My gratitude begins with my first friend in the cancer world: Irene Ydens. Thank you for your friendship, for knowing I needed help, and for your unwavering advocacy for all children. Luke was lucky to have you as a mama, as I am to have you as my friend. You taught me I had options and how to rally for my baby.

Thank you to my film acting coach, Deb Fink, at the American Conservatory Theater in San Francisco, who spotted something in a piece I wrote in 2020 about cancer and asked me pointedly,

"What was THAT about? There's something big here!" You made me realize it was time to set this story free.

Thank you to my lifelong buddy, Alicia, for listening to my story about this crazy experience in film acting class and reminding me that one of our mutual childhood theater friends was now a huge player in the book-birthing business. A new connection was made!

Thank you, Linda Sivertsen, the Book Mama, for leading me to your amazing online book proposal course. It gave me direction, purpose, and inspiration. Your smarts, kindness, advice, and introductions led me to the next person on this journey.

Allison Lane, the incredible editing, writing, and marketing guru of Allison Lane Literary. From day one, you have been my person, bringing my book proposal to life. You challenged me to be better every step of the way with your extraordinary prowess and insights. You are the best cheerleader a girl could want, and you kept me motivated, focused, and proud of the work. I'm so grateful for your smarts and, mostly, for how deeply you care. Because of you, I was introduced to Linda Stirling, my now publisher!

Linda, I am eternally honored that you chose me to be a part of The Publishing Circle family. Your belief in me and the importance of this project has made it all happen. You are a constant source of inspiration, with a healthy dose of reality and calm. I'm eternally grateful for your tenacity, creativity, and perfectionism in getting it all just right. You are an amazing publisher who truly hears an author's story and collaborates beautifully.

I had the most incredible contributors and early readers, many of whom were from our cancer years at Lucile Packard Children's Hospital at Stanford! It was a full-circle experience working with them on this book.

Thank you to our incredible oncologist, Dr. Gary Dahl, for giving our child her health and well-being and for leading such a kick-ass medical team. It's been somewhat surreal and incredibly empowering to have your generous support through this process all these years later. Eternal gratitude also goes to our talented and kind nurse practitioner, Stacey Teicher, who always has the best advice, whether caring so compassionately for Cecilia twenty-five years ago or recently with all your help on the manuscript. Thank you for allowing me to interview you and for sharing your sage and meaningful thoughts. My gratitude to Pam Simon, an incredible nurse and program director for the AYA center and a tireless networker for me. Your support has meant the world!

Thank you to Khim Choong, MSTCM, L. Ac., ACN, and Dan Labriola, ND, and Doni Wilson ND for sharing your knowledge and passion for complementary medicine. You made an enormous difference in Cecilia's cancer experience and mine as a caregiver.

To Dr. Stephanie Smith, my soul sister in survivorship advocacy! It is incredible to work with you on various projects and have your contribution to the survivorship chapter. Your research and advocacy for families is changing the world of childhood cancer.

To my first readers: Dr. Gary Dahl; Stacey Teicher, NP; Dr. Stephanie Smith; Pam Simon, MSN, CPP, CPON; Dr. Brooke Vittimberga, and parents Jill Whisler, Jean Cripps, Sam Taylor, and Fatima Khoogar. What a labor of love! Thank you for reading the first draft and providing me with insightful notes and directions for refining and making *The Cancer Parent's Handbook* relatable to all.

Thank you to Lucile Packard Children's Hospital for all of your support for *The Cancer Parent's Handbook* and for taking such loving care of us throughout our daughter's treatment. We are forever indebted to everyone at LPCH. We were lucky to live near Jacob's Heart Cancer Supportive Services, who provided our entire family with both a mental and physical outlet for our fear and grief—and a whole lot of fun, all under the leadership of Lori Butterworth and her incredible staff.

To the fearless parents in the Facebook groups for childhood cancers 2020-2025, thank you for allowing me to ask you endless questions, for your wise feedback, and for your contribution to *The Cancer Parent's Handbook*.

We were blessed to have some incredible people by our side during our journey, and I never lose sight of that privilege.

To Joni, our magical caregiver, who always found a way for Cecilia to play and be a child amidst the worst of her trauma. Thank you for giving her the power of her spirit animal: dinos!!! And thank you for your gentle, loving care for Madi while her sister was in treatment.

To all our family, friends, and work colleagues who lifted us up for years, and a special shout out to "Mama Nikki," who knew when to show up, get stuff done, and be present. I'll never forget. Thank you to my siblings, Lynn, Leighanne, and Glenn, who although far away, always kept us close in so many ways.

Thank you to my big sis, Leighanne, for pushing me towards this project and helping me to find my light.

We were so lucky to have all four grandparents in the neighborhood when cancer struck our little family. To Pauline, Glenn, Marie, and Nils, thank you for using your strengths and superpowers to keep our family afloat. You were everything to us, not only tactically but emotionally as well. Thank you for your strength and love. To my parents, Pauline and Glenn, a special thank you for being my guiding light and shining example of how to love hard, protect fiercely, and give abundantly. I feel you guiding me every day.

Thank you to my girlfriends (you know who you are), near and far, for keeping me steady and sane, cheering me on, and helping in so many ways, big and small. I love you!

And to my family—where to begin? When I think of our little family now and then, I'm so proud of us and how we've loved together, grown together, and are having so much fun together now as grown-ups! I couldn't imagine another group better equipped to fiercely love, nurture, and grow as we live life together and thrive. We. Are. Family!

To Madi and Ellie:

Madi, thank you for insisting that you be a part of everything during your "is's" treatment years. You showed us that family being together is a must during a crisis. And you showered us endlessly with your toddler sunshine therapy and were the most compassionate sibling and buddy ever.

To our "baby" Ellie, bringing you into the world right after treatment was nothing but joy and love. You brought so much laughter and light to our family then and continue to bring so much light now as you perfectly completed our little family at a crucial transition in our lives.

Thank you both for your spot-on notes for the book, your moral support, and endless cheerleading.

Cecilia, our little warrior (now badass woman). The way you processed and continue to process your treatment years after the trauma that comes from over 2,000 needle pokes and endless prods is remarkable. You were the most incredible little four-year-old patient, with a fierceness and hilarity that made this journey doable as you brightened the days of every doctor and nurse at LPCH. You showered us with your devotion, love, and complete trust, even on the scariest of days. You are a tribute to all warrior kids. Thank you for helping me tell not only my story but your story for the benefit of countless children who will be diagnosed with cancer every year. And to my lover, boyfriend, sweetheart, my hubby, Arne. I always knew I won the lottery when I met you, and this entire journey has proven that to be true. You have been a constant advocate for this project, nudging me toward doing it and encouraging me every step to dive deeper, go further, and advocate harder for the countless families who need it. You are the consummate (and most annoying) editor ever and were instrumental in helping me stay true to my voice and our experience. Thank you for being willing to help in so many ways, big and small, and for being my person. I am the luckiest girl in the world.

Contents

the Cancer Parent's Handbook

What Your Oncologist Doesn't Have Time To Tell You

"Everyone needs help along the way.
You'll get that in *The Cancer Parent's Handbook*.
I don't think I've ever seen anything like this in any book."
GARY DAHL, MD, Pediatric Oncology

LAURA DeKRAKER LANG-REE

the publishing CIRCLE.

A Note to Readers

I want you to know that I see you, feel you, and know your pain. Although my time as a cancer-warrior mama has passed, the sense of where you are today is always fresh in my heart because as cancer parents, we are part of a lifelong club now—and we get it. Even if our children survive, each time we hear about another diagnosis or see a sweet bald-headed child, we take a deep breath and remember, oh so clearly, what it's like to be right where you are now.

This book was lovingly created for you, based on my experiences and the observations of so many other people I've met over the years, including a wonderful cohort of current warrior parents who volunteered their thoughts and perspectives. This book is meant to represent as many of us as possible, because cancer doesn't discriminate. Some of us have extended families, others are alone. Some may have money to spare, and others barely enough to scrape by, much less handle the financial strain of cancer. Some of us have a partner, and others deal with cancer as a solo parent.

Despite our differences, we are united in one thing—saving our child. The tools and tips in *The Cancer Parent's Handbook* are designed for all of you with love and care, regardless of your circumstance. So, as you read, find what works for you and disregard the rest. Or let something inspire you to create your own amazing solutions.

With love,
Laura

Foreword

If you're reading this, it's likely you or someone you love is facing a dire and heartbreaking challenge: a child's cancer diagnosis. Please know you have my utmost compassion. My heart goes out to you, your family, and that precious child. My hope is for a complete recovery.

This book is for you. It was lovingly conceived, researched, and written by cancer mom Laura DeKraker Lang-Ree, whose daughter Cecilia was a patient of mine.

I chose to study and practice pediatrics, specifically pediatric oncology, because of the opportunity to provide care for a whole family going through that experience, as well as that specialty gave me a chance to make a difference where it was most needed.

When I began seeing childhood cancer patients over fifty years ago, I rarely had good news for families. That drove me to want to be a part of what has become a tremendous medical success story. Beginning with my twelve years at St. Jude Children's Research Hospital, and now my nearly thirty-five years here at Lucile Packard Children's Hospital Stanford, I've witnessed a dramatic rise in long-term survivorship from childhood cancers over those decades. This is thanks to tireless and dedicated work by countless researchers, doctors, nurses, and donors, to name a few. I am deeply grateful for the opportunity to have contributed to that.

However, for families facing a diagnosis today, the personal experience, from the paralyzing terror of the initial diagnosis to the bewildering and numbing grind of a lengthy treatment protocol remains much the same. We doctors give parents the detailed lowdown on their child's treatment plan and focus on the patient's medical care. Overwhelmed, parents are left to navigate everything else on their own. This book sets out to change that.

Having treated something like 1,500 childhood cancer patients in my career, of course I don't remember every family. Laura DeKraker Lang-Ree, along with her husband, Arne, and their warrior daughter, Cecilia, I remember very well. A fierce advocate for her daughter's care and cure, Laura left no question unanswered, no option unexplored in her relentless pursuit of the best experience possible for Cecilia.

Cecilia was a precocious four-year-old, always ready with a knock-knock joke for me, her hospital room decked out in her favorite themes, and always looking for me to blow up a purple glove balloon. She was tough, too, lovingly coached by her parents to take all the pokes and prods in stride. How delighted I was, then, to meet up with Cecilia many years later—by then an undergrad here at Stanford—when she invited me to speak to a group of students at a cancer fundraising event she organized.

You now hold in your hands a manual for how Laura made sure Cecilia got the best care possible, both from the medical team here at Stanford and from other wellness practitioners. Backed by Laura's relentless research, and a deep commitment to loving parenting, *The Cancer Parent's Handbook* brings together a wealth of knowledge, experience, and information so you can give your child the very best nutritional, physical, emotional, and mental support possible.

With a pragmatic and approachable style, Laura is your navigator, coach, companion, and confidant, from diagnosis and the chaotic early days of treatment, through inpatient stays and outpatient treatments, to family life at home with a childhood cancer patient. With detailed lists, abundant references, and great ideas for dealing with a host of challenges, Laura lights the way to help you advocate effectively for your child's care while tending to your own well-being as well as the emotional health of your family.

The goals are simple and are the same for every family facing childhood cancer: do everything you can with the things you can control to support your child's health while helping your family thrive and making sure your kid has every opportunity to just be a kid.

This last point is one of the most important pieces of advice I can give you from my five decades on the oncology wards—try as best you can to normalize what you are now facing. Live life as if cancer is just one part of it, not as if this experience is separate from the rest of your life. As impossible as that might sound, it is doable. Take a deep breath, turn the page, and let Laura show you how.

I am privileged to recommend this book to families facing the daunting challenges, and thrilled knowing more and more parents will now have *The Cancer Parent's Handbook* within reach during such trying times.

All of my best wishes for health and recovery to you and your child.

Dr. Gary Dahl
Pediatric Oncology & Hematology, Lucile Packard Children's Hospital at Stanford
Professor Emeritus, Stanford University Medicine
Architect, The Health After Treatment (HAT) Program at Lucile Packard

1

Through the Fire
There's a Dragon at the Gate

There is a dragon at the gate who means to do your child harm. Raise the drawbridge. Polish your armor. Sharpen your swords. You will find a way to fight and defeat it. The stakes are too high to do anything less than everything you can. A time will come to take off your armor and breathe again, and you will be the hope for another family.

I WROTE THAT LITTLE STORY DURING MY FIVE-YEAR JOURNEY with childhood cancer—my child's cancer treatment. Cecilia was diagnosed with ALL, acute lymphoblastic leukemia, when she was just three-and-a-half years old. Right now, you are reading this because somebody, your child, or a child you love, has been given a horrific and lengthy diagnosis like Cecilia was given— childhood cancer—and it sucks.

The idea of cancer choosing my daughter, our family, my life, left me speechless. Maybe you're speechless right now, too. It also left me pissed off and made me become a fierce warrior for my daughter, our family, and myself.

Cecilia is one of the lucky ones. She survived.

I know that's your number one hope—that your child survives, and that life can get back to some kind of "normal." Maybe you've already done a little light Google searching on your child's form of cancer. Not fun, is it? Yes, cancer survival rates have improved across the board, yet the incidence of childhood cancer has continued to increase over the last thirty years. Wow.

The good news is this: about eighty percent of children diagnosed with cancer today survive. Let that really sink in—eighty percent— and compare that to children in the 50s, 60s, and 70s. About half of them died. This is thanks to the incredible work by oncologists, nurses, and researchers worldwide. I am eternally grateful to our oncology team, because I know first-hand what amazing work they did for our child and so many more.

If you are like me, you realize that an eighty percent survival rate is something to be grateful for. But it really didn't make me happy. The number of kids that still die today overall—fifteen percent— or who are left with life-altering side effects from the drugs that cure them, is far too high. The thought that one of those might be Cecilia pissed me off, too, and put me on a mission to help parents like us not just survive this cancer expedition we've been forced to take but come out on the other side intact. Maybe even stronger as a person, tighter as a family, empowered and determined to find a new chapter once your child is cured. That feeling, that anger, that mission, became the fuel for this book.

I began taking notes over twenty-four years ago during Cecilia's treatment when I realized there was no guidebook to help me. Yes, there was a protocol for the medicine that would hopefully let her be one of the survivors, and one book geared towards the medical side of treatment (which I was very grateful for), but there wasn't significant information for everything else, including what I could do to contribute to her cure, and to her daily life during treatment.

- No book with suggestions and advice on how to keep my family intact during this crisis.
- No toolbox for learning how to ask for help from my loving friends and family who were at a loss for what to do.
- No handbook for how to talk to our medical team and become a collaborator.
- No resource about how to manage the fear and anxiety surrounding a child's life-threatening illness.

What did I want? I wanted help. I wanted one book with all that information and more from somebody who'd been there, done that, and who had lots of expert advice to share.

It didn't exist. So, twenty-four years later, I made it happen.

The Freakout

Our story began when I realized we were facing at least two-and-a-half years of treatment, and two-and-a-half years of follow-up care—if we were lucky. Here's what I initially thought: There's no freaking way . . .

> *What if she dies???*
>
> *How am I going to make it to the end?*
>
> *What if she dies!!!*
>
> *How was Cecilia's fifteen-month-old sister going to handle this?*
>
> *What if she dies?*
>
> *How am I going to handle this?*
>
> *What if she dies!*
>
> *What if my husband and I get divorced from all the stress?*

WHAT IF SHE DIES . . .

What about the plans for my life, my career, my family?

Living in this constant spiral of emotions began to burn me up and burn me out. Fear, debilitating anxiety, rage, lack of sleep, and confusion, became my constant companions as these draining thoughts, and so many more, took hold in my mind. You too? I totally get it. These kinds of thoughts are natural when a crisis starts, so don't punish yourself for having them. But have you also noticed how unhelpful they are?

One thing I felt shortly after diagnosis was that I didn't want to be, couldn't be, angry, sad, and anxiety-fueled for five freakin' years. I wouldn't survive.

My sweet baby showed me the way out.

> *"Positude", a word coined by our three-year-old daughter, Cecilia, a few weeks into treatment for acute lymphoblastic leukemia.*

Positude to the Rescue

"Positude", a word coined by our three-year-old daughter, Cecilia, a few weeks into treatment for acute lymphoblastic leukemia. One day, Arne and I were prepping Cecilia, doing our best to get her psyched up for yet another injection—over 2,000 in total for her protocol. As I laid out the agenda for the day, including the necessary procedures, on a whim (or maybe it was a fabulous parenting moment) I decided to include all the positive aspects as well. A playdate afterward, the promise of a popsicle for being polite and kind to the oncologists and nurses, and practicing her "whale breathing", her version of Lamaze, as she was injected once again. After our lengthy description of the day's events and hearing our request to "have a positive attitude", she declared with excitement, "You mean a *Positude!*"

Positude became our mantra. Our rallying cry! It was empowering for Cecilia. A focal point for us as her parents. Something for our family to strive for as we pushed through the fire.

Positude, amidst the chaos and the fear, gently shifted our focus toward finding the light—every day.

The idea of striving for a positive attitude during trauma isn't new and it certainly was not something we came up with on our own during treatment. We were lucky enough to be shown pivotal examples of how a positive mindset makes a huge difference in a child's day from our wonderful oncologist, Dr. Gary Dahl, our skilled nurse practitioner, Stacey, the kind nurses administering chemo (especially our favorites Melissa and Leslie), other parents, online support buddies, and our beloved Jacob's Heart Children's Cancer Center.

All of that shaped how we decided to set the tone for the next two-and-a-half years and the routines and rituals we created around each day in that marathon. Ideas and strategies were shared with us. We shared them with others and created a way of being during treatment that got us through the fire and slayed that dragon for good. The decision to focus on the positive using concrete strategies and tactics to advocate for our very lives made an enormous difference in our family's mental and physical outcome. I'm sure of it.

The Cancer Parent's Handbook will help you find your Positude. It's really not enough to say, "Look at the bright side!" or "You'll get through this!" which is often what friends and family say to help you, and themselves, feel better. You are in the zone. You need specific tactics and techniques you can apply right now to whatever phase you find yourself in with your child, and *The Cancer Parent's Handbook* will show you how. Steal my exact suggestions (I'd love that!) or let them be a catalyst for you to come up with something even better that makes your life, and your child's life, as strong, resilient, and positive as it can be—now, and always.

Not feeling terribly positive right now? I truly get it. That's why I'm here to help you. I have the perspective of time, and I'm fiercely armed with compassion, wisdom, and strong tactics and strategies for cancer parents. I'll help you to wrap your head around your crisis and intentionally create your new normal with tested strategies and actionable tactics for each and every phase of treatment and follow-up care. But for a moment, let's pause and reflect on what you've just been through, those things that are common for every parent whose child has been diagnosed with cancer. And it all begins with diagnosis.

D-Day

Diagnosis day. A day forever imprinted in your soul. "D-Day" in our house: January 6th, 1999.

For weeks, something was off. Our bouncy, energetic little girl was lethargic, asking to be picked up constantly, and her skin was growing increasingly pale.

At the park, a place she adored, she couldn't even manage to do more than sit and pick grass, then asked to be picked up. She didn't have any interest in the swings or the slide. No interest in anything besides being held. By the time I got home, her lips were blue. I took her inside to warm her up in a sink-bath and nudged Arne, saying, "Doesn't she look pale to you?"

"I'm not sure," he replied.

Both of us wanted to live in denial a little longer. After all, she didn't have a fever, cough, or runny nose. She was fine, right? Dear God, right?

But I knew something wasn't right. So did she.

At bedtime, I asked her point blank, "Where does it hurt, baby?" She rubbed her torso and said simply, "Everywhere, Mama."

The next day, I insisted that our doctor run labs—something they didn't think necessary. But I knew better. That was the beginning of my transformation into being a fierce advocate for my child, and I didn't even realize it. Arne came with me for the check-up and blood draw. Somehow, we both knew that shit was about to hit the fan.

I'll never forget that wash of shock, fear, and utter paralysis a few hours later when our daughter's pediatrician called Arne at home with the news: Cecilia had leukemia. Shit indeed.

I'm a teacher and I was mid-class, teaching a show-choir some new dance moves. Of course, I'd been worried about the labs and the results. But never did I think the word cancer would come out of my husband's mouth when he reached me at work. I felt like all my students' eyes were on me as I desperately tried to keep it together in front of them.

I ran to the front office to quickly tell my principals that something was terribly wrong, that I was leaving campus indefinitely. Meanwhile, Arne was at home with Cecilia, trying not to cry. The orders? Get to Clinic D ASAP, the cancer ward at Lucile Packard Children's Hospital.

Within the hour, one of our best friends, Nikki, along with our parents, who lived in the area, swarmed the house to prepare us for heading into the fire. My head spun. On the one hand, I was trying to be strong for Cecilia; on the other, I was falling apart in front of the people who loved me the most.

Leaving a bewildered baby Madi, just fifteen months old, in the arms of her bestemor (grandma, in Norwegian) my heart broke as I looked over my shoulder, the front door closing.

Arne and I headed to Clinic D, which would become our new home away from home, where a waiting room full of sweet kids with bald heads whose sympathetic eyes met ours as they quickly assessed us as another new case. Even at that moment, part of me still clung to a notion that we didn't belong there; the upcoming tests would surely reveal it was all a big mistake.

Sound familiar? I was not ready.

Ready Or Not

As much as you want to crawl back under the blankets after diagnosis day, life in the childhood cancer world quickly demands that you wake up, pay close attention, and become organized and knowledgeable as you ready yourself to take on the role of the advocate and gatekeeper for your child's treatment years and follow-up care. Nobody tells you this is what you've signed up for— at least not in the medical community. Armed with good instincts, a pile of cancer books I frantically bought online (only one focused on the medical side of childhood cancer), and shared wisdom from an incredible bevy of cancer warrior parents I found online and at our clinic, I slowly uncovered the truth: there is no roadmap for parenting a kid with cancer. That realization is paralyzing at least, overwhelming at best.

We were admitted that afternoon and settled in for . . . what? We didn't know. Days? Weeks? You know the drill from your own D-Day, as it all depends on your child's state when they enter the hospital and how they react to the first round of treatment. I know families who spent the first month of treatment in-patient. Talk about going through the fire from day one!

Cecilia got "lucky", spending "only" five days in the hospital where she received her diagnostic spinal tap and a bag of blood from her bestefar (grandfather) which she sorely needed as the leukemia made her as white as a sheet. Watching that blood do its work, and the pink return to her cheeks, was a gift, taking the edge off my panic for a moment. Then, suddenly, the nurse handed over her discharge papers, chemo schedule, and said brightly, "You've got this now!"

Huh? Are you kidding me? It sure didn't feel like I got it. Cue tears and full-on freak out as I realized, holy crap, this is up to us. Deep breath.

Here's what I didn't know then: you don't need to know everything or do everything on day one. Or even month one.

As a parent of a newly diagnosed child, you can only absorb a limited amount of what's happening each moment, much less years from now. That's perfectly normal. You and your child are both scared of this diagnosis and the sudden onslaught of needles and medicine. You are in fight-or-flight mode and maybe some lingering denial. It's tempting to get defensive, to question everything the medical team needs to do. For the moment, though, you need to trust they know what they're doing because they do—they are the experts. The early weeks of treatment are normally standardized anyway, with very few decisions for you to make, so you don't need to worry about the details of the process quite yet. You just need to focus on your child.

> People shut off when their child gets sick. Parents don't talk, kids don't either. I encourage parents to try to forget about the disease—live! Doctors and nurses take care of that part of the disease. A parent's job is to be present... to have fun.
>
> **—DR. GARY DAHL**

Your baby needs to know you are right there with them, loving them deeply, and keeping them calm, and infusing a bit of fun and silly into even their darkest days. I guarantee they are more scared and confused than you and need more than anything the affirmation that you will stay by their side, together in the eye of this hurricane. And, as Dr. Dahl suggests, fun can and will return to your life— even during treatment.

2

What You Need to Know Right Now

What you need to know for the first few weeks of treatment was gathered from a combination of my own notes from our treatment years, as well as bits of wisdom from other warrior parents that we met along the way. As the parent of a newly diagnosed child, you have some time to catch your breath. Then we'll look at what's next.

What You Need to Know Right Now – The Big Picture

- Stay centered
  Breathe deeply. You are surrounded by really smart oncologists and nurses, and your child will probably be assigned to a well-tested protocol. If there are big decisions to make, they will tell you. Otherwise, this initial time is fairly cookie-cutter.

- Surrender to what is: your child has cancer

  This is a biggie. I'm not saying give up—but surrender. There is a huge difference. When you can accept what is happening, you can move forward. In the beginning, you'll need to breathe a lot and surrender again and again. Not to fear; you will learn how to surrender in upcoming chapters.

- Keep it simple

  Come up with a simple, age-appropriate, and non-terrifying way to explain what's going on to your child. For our almost four-year-old we said, "You know how you have not been feeling so great? We found out the problem (name it)! And you are going to get help now."

- Document everything

  You are in crisis mode, so don't rely on your memory to help you right now. Bring a notebook or laptop and/or record all meetings with your medical team. If possible, bring your spouse, partner, or a friend to these meetings so you have help hearing and absorbing information. This is key because your brain is full of worry right now, and hearing what's being said can be challenging. If you can't bring a buddy, voice record the meeting on your phone.

What You Need to Know Right Now – Friends, Family, School, and Work

- Seek help with sending updates

  Ask one good friend or family member to text or email those nearest and dearest with an update. And remember, no guilt if you forget someone. They will understand.

- Inform school

  Have that same friend call school for all your children and fill them in. Your kids will not be doing much homework this week, maybe not the next. Eventually, you'll come up with a schedule for your school-aged kids who are in treatment. For now, homework doesn't matter (I say this as a teacher!).

- Accept help from friends and family!
  Whether it's someone to sit with your child so you can put your face in the sun and cry, financial help, food, a drop-off of clothing or a walk, you need the help. Take it. In later chapters I'll teach you how to make all the offers of help work for you, and if you are not getting those offers, how to ask for them. You don't know who will step up to help you and your family. Sometimes this fight is too much for people you'd expect to be by your side. Sometimes it's the unexpected person who runs along with you. Accept whatever is offered.

- Explore other networks of help
  If you are not near family or friends, talk to your social worker and Child Life Services to see what their volunteers can help you with at home, or while in the hospital. If you are part of a religious community, let the office know what's up, asap.

- Contact HR
  If employed, call HR and let them know what's happening. Find out your rights around taking time off.

What You Need to Know Right Now – Medically

- Never be afraid to ask questions. In fact, ask your doctor to repeat themselves often.
  At least once a day, your oncologist will come by to update you and chat. Step out of the room and into the hallways when your medical team arrives so you can be vulnerable and real without worrying about your child. You will have big, scary questions to ask your oncologist,

and your child *does not benefit from seeing your fear*. It just freaks them out.

You will have time later to figure out how you want to talk with your kid about treatment duration and what's to come, so pace yourself. Later, especially if your child is older, they may want to be a part of these daily hospital chats from your oncologist so they can also ask questions and feel that their voice is being heard.

Insist that your care team listens to you and treats the whole child, not just their cancer. All your questions and concerns are valid.

- Center your child
  When the nurse or phlebotomist comes into your room, ask for details about what they need to do and insist they give you the time and space to center your child. Then, ask your child if they want you to hold their hand or cuddle—whatever provides comfort and gives them some agency. Nobody wants to get randomly stuck with a needle without warning.

- Speak up
  You know your child better than the doctors and nurses, so if you feel like something isn't right, it probably isn't. Report any change in behavior, look, or mood, as nine times out of ten you will be right, and something will be wrong. Doctors and nurses rely on you to spot things because you know your kid best. I realize this is freaking terrifying right now, but you can do it. Trust your instincts, observe, and report. Never shy away from speaking up.

- Check everything (twice)
  Always, always ask your nurse to double-check medications before they're administered—and have them teach you how to verify the bags or bottles yourself.

You're the parent, which means you're now part of the quality control team. Check the medication and blood type labels every single time, ensuring that the medicine and blood type are correct, and, most importantly, has your child's name on them. As surprising as it sounds, it is ultimately your responsibility to ensure the medicine is for your child, that it is the correct medication, and that it is administered at the right time. Nobody else will do this for you.

- Get smart
  Study your treatment plan (often called the roadmap or care plan). Understand the treatment as best as you can. Your growing wisdom may shock the crap out of your doctors, but it will also help you know what's coming up and what to expect. Right now, just study the treatment plan so you can ask initial questions. Later, you can dig deeper.

- Connect with your medical team
  Strive to find a good connection with your medical team, but if it's just not clicking, it's okay to request a new oncologist. Your child will be with them for years to come, so that positive connection is important. But do give it time to evolve before deciding to switch.

- Meet your social worker
  Introduce yourself to the hospital social worker. Next month, you can ask for help with both small and large financial issues.

What You Need to Know Right Now – You & Your Child

- Avoid overindulging
  Do your best to limit the treats, junk food, excess gifts, or toys. It will be tempting to ply them with donuts and Legos because they have to get an IV, or if they won't

eat. But in the long run, this will be a difficult habit to unwind.

- Set boundaries
Continue expecting the manners and kindness your child has been taught. Unless they are a puddle of tears, let them know that please, thank you, and kindness are still part of your family drill.

- Avoid comparisons
Every child's journey is different. What happens to someone else's child doesn't mean it will happen to yours.

- Focus on yourself
Your mental health is paramount. If you are not okay, nobody is. There will be hard days, but there will also be many silver linings. Look for them and hold on to them tightly. Take this day by day, moment by moment, and try not to worry about what might be, just about what is (surrender!). It's okay to feel joy in the beginning, even when everything is scary. Intentionally bring as much joy in as possible.

- Nix perfectionism
You don't owe anyone anything right now. Just focus on your children, your partner, and the people who are of genuine help. You don't have to talk to or see anyone who is draining you, no matter what their relationship is to you/your child.

- Remember your partner
If you are in a relationship, prioritize it because if you don't, it could fall apart. And if you are handling this solo, prioritize yourself. Right now, keep it simple. Find times for rest, short walks, and some alone time to process what's happening.

- One day at a time
  Take things one day at a time, sometimes one hour at a time. Each day may look different, and inconsistency is part of this journey, especially right now. In a few weeks or months, a routine will be established, and we'll talk about how to manage those times in The New Normal chapter.

- Breathe
  Someday, this will all be a memory.

  When I asked my husband why our daughter was the one who had cancer and why couldn't I take on the burden for her, he said, "She has the best chance of beating this. If one of us were to take this on, she would more than likely have to grow up without one of us." Satisfied with his answer, I then asked him if I could at least take on her pain. He said, "No, she needs to feel the pain, so she knows when to fight."

  I have reminded myself of this countless times over the last two years. We celebrated her freedom from chemo last week.

  —RINDI AND MATTHEW, CANCER PARENTS

For most families, that's all you need to think about for the time being. However, there are cases where you must make big decisions quickly, so stay alert and ask questions.

We had to make critical decisions about the route of treatment in the first few days of his diagnosis. Decisions had to be made quickly due to a fast-growing tumor in the eye. As our heads were spinning and still in shock, we had to also hear and weigh in on the pros and cons of treatment for a disease we knew nothing about.

—FATIMA, CANCER MOM

If you can only focus on one thing, focus on yourself and your child, accept what is, and remember to be present. The following chapters spell out what can wait, and what's to come as you move past the diagnosis phase.

3

What Can Wait

I N THE FIRST FEW WEEKS, IT'S TEMPTING TO THINK YOU NEED to know everything. You don't. *The Cancer Parent's Handbook* is filled with chapters devoted to each aspect of life in the cancer world, and guides you, with Toolbox Tips, on how to effectively manage your situation.

For right now, here is a list of things you can wait to think about until after the initial phase of treatment has passed, which is typically a month in. It's good to know what's coming.

Coming Soon (Just Not Yet)

- Becoming the expert about your child's cancer
- A full nutrition plan for the family
- A reward system for regular treatment days (early weeks are not regular or normal)
- Establishing a routine for regular chemo days in the maintenance part of treatment

- Meeting the hospital social worker to talk about financial options both big and small

- Meeting the hospital child life specialist and learning about all of their wonderful activities both in the room and at the hospital

- Individual therapy

- Regular mental health checks for you from a professional

- Boundary setting with your medical team, friends, and family about how they engage with you and your child about treatment

- Boundary setting with your friends and family about how and when they can visit (just don't have them visit for now, while Absolute Neutrophil Count (or ANC) is low)

- Creating an easy way to update people

- Developing a plan for extended help. For now, just say yes. You are going to need help for years.

- A plan for schoolwork and homework. Give it a few weeks.

- A plan for how you want to talk to your child about treatment overall

- Options in your protocol for treatment timing and location (i.e., local labs vs hospital)

- Creating a plan for understanding and proactively working through side effects, both short and long term

- Adding complementary therapies to the protocol

- Regular self-care and date nights

- Establishing new family routines and finding fun again

I know this list of what's coming soon is daunting, which is one of the many reasons I wrote this book. Not to worry. I will take you step by step through each one of them and give you the tools you need to not just survive your child's treatment, but thrive. Let's get started by looking at how *The Cancer Parent's Handbook* is organized.

Developing Your Toolbox—What To Expect

Chapter by chapter, I'll share what to expect and how to navigate through each phase of a typical treatment process (one without recurrence) with grace, strategy, and smarts. I'm blessed to collaborate in *The Cancer Parent's Handbook* with brilliant oncologists, nurses, and natural health experts who share their wisdom about side effects, strengthening your child's immune system without getting in the way of treatment, and how parents can become true partners in their child's care.

I began writing *The Cancer Parent's Handbook* during our treatment years as I accumulated tips and tricks from those fabulous professionals as well as therapists, support groups, nurses, fellow parents, copious reading, and our own trial and error. I shared them with every new parent I met online and in the hospital via email and colorful flyers. Back then, I regularly declared, "I have a book in me." But it took time, a lot of healing, and a fresh perspective for me to be ready to go back into those dark years and bring a sense of power to give to you, the parents whose child has been newly diagnosed.

You need a road map for all the questions and situations that will come up:

- How can I get my child to swallow their chemo pill?
- What can I do to stop my baby from screaming during her injections?
- Is there any way to make a hospital visit less scary?
- What about processing chemo? Can she play? Go to school?
- How can I get my partner/friends/family to help out?

There are proven tools to help answer these questions, and effective strategies that show you ways to create your team so you don't have to do this alone. Until now, that information has been scattered to the wind in random sources, making it impossible to wrap your head around the big picture of living with cancer. That's why each chapter covers a specific topic from diagnosis through follow-up treatment and is loaded with Toolbox Tips and advice for every step.

What's A Toolbox Tip?

In each chapter, we'll discuss a topic in depth, options for your family, and any expert advice. Toolbox Tips give you direct and detailed tips for how to gracefully and wisely handle life with cancer. They are sprinkled all over the chapters of *The Cancer Parent's Handbook*. Maybe you've just gotten the diagnosis; maybe you are already well into the trenches. Either way, step one is getting organized and knowledgeable about your child's protocol. This next chapter gives you the strategies to do just that.

> 💡 **Toolbox Tip:**
> Decide the best way for you to get and stay organized. Consider setting up a Google folder or hit your local or online bookstore for a journal. Find one format to use and stick to it. Do this right away and then, let's get going.

Hold your child close, love your partner with ferocity, reach out and truly lean on those friends and family who are showing up for you right this minute. They want to be useful, to run alongside you on this journey—that's why they are showing up.

Reflect on these beautiful words as we move forward, from a wise cancer mom who is currently in the trenches:

> *This is not your fault. It's okay to cry, to feel sad, angry, and every other emotion. I know at the beginning it is hard to just think about the next five minutes and we wanna know what's gonna happen. It's tough not to know. But your own baby is gonna make you stronger every time you see them and even with all that is happening, they still have a smile for you. That makes everything worth it. That is gonna give you the energy you need to keep going.* —**CANDY, CANCER MOM**

4

Get Your Shit Together

Knowledge is Power (and so is a spreadsheet).

LAURA DEKRAKER LANG-REE

After the first month of treatment, if we are lucky, things settle down and become more routine. It's time to get your shit together for the long haul.

Starting this part of your child's cancer journey can feel a lot like being thrown into the wilderness without a map. You don't have a choice, it looks pretty damn scary, and you know for sure what you want at the end of the trip—to get out with your child cured.

Gut-wrenching fear is pervasive in these early weeks as you learn about your child's diagnosis, staging, treatment, and imminent hospital stays as the cancer is, hopefully, pushed into remission. This is normal. You've gone through a powerful shock. Acknowledging that fear is essential in order to move through the trauma. Only then can you take those first steps towards getting informed and organized and take action against this fear in a constructive and positive way. It's time to stop spiraling and move towards more constructive thinking.

Here's how: Become the expert.

Knowledge is power, helping to deflect that pervasive fear that comes with a cancer diagnosis. If you want to be a part of your child's medical team instead of a frantic bystander, you need to be the #1 expert in all things cancer as your child begins this next phase of treatment. This is a job title nobody tells you about in the beginning. And because you are overwhelmed by the diagnosis, and cancer is high stakes, it's easy to initially fall into the trap of thinking that the cure lies entirely with your oncologist and nurses. Not true. These amazing people have a lot on their plates, first and foremost establishing the proper diagnosis for your child and making sure the treatment schedule is set. The rest, my friends, is up to us.

Fear and panic are exacerbated by a lack of knowledge, especially right now. I bet you recognize that cold fact. Change that narrative by getting informed, learning the ropes, and fully understanding what this marathon you've been thrust into will be like as the days, months and years play out. Sounds like work? It is. But the payoff is enormous. Being knowledgeable about your child's treatment helps you to fill in the blanks, ask relevant questions, make meaningful choices, and imagine a future where you'll have the power to show up for whatever you may face.

The following are action items for the early weeks.

Build Your Knowledge Base

Step one is building your knowledge base, so read as much as you can about your child's cancer. See what information your medical team has to give you, purchase books online (set a budget so you are not tempted to overspend), or hit up your local library or the hospital library to see what resources they have for cancer in general, as well as your child's cancer. See Resources for examples of cancer books you can purchase.

💡 Toolbox Tip:

Order a mix of books to give you a broader perspective and knowledge base on cancer in general and your child's cancer, in particular, if books specifically about it exist. They do tend to be fairly medical in nature, so choose carefully so you are not overwhelmed.

There are some wonderful children's books about cancer that can really help a child process what they are going through. Our favorite was *The Jester Has Lost His Jingle!*

Another option for getting smart(er) is to join a support group of parents whose children have the same diagnosis. Their knowledge and ability to teach you the ropes is invaluable. You will learn things from other parents who are slightly ahead of you in treatment that is just not available or shared at the hospital—how to take a particular medicine, reactions to chemo, and ways to circumvent feeling lousy after a treatment. Pure gold.

Make Friends

Finding new friends that understand what you are going through is a huge way to build your knowledge base. Online parent cancer groups are amazing at sharing resources, opinions, and knowledge, and members provide a healthy dose of love and cheerleading when needed. They are a lifeline.

Here's a list of a few Facebook groups for some common cancers. Some are disease specific, and some are more general cancer advice and support groups. If you don't see your child's cancer below, a quick Google search will help you find online support quickly.

- Childhood Acute Lymphoblastic Leukemia
- Momcology
- Families of Childhood Cancer Support Group
- Neuroblastoma Family Support Group

A longer list of cancer parent groups and family support groups is provided in Resources.

> ### 💡 Toolbox Tip:
>
> Set a limit on the time spent on research and knowledge building. Time spent researching can become obsessive, then overwhelming. Figure out what feels like too much for you, set some boundaries, and then walk away and pet your cat, take a walk, go outside and put your face in the sun. You need the balance of living in cancer vs. living with cancer. My rule of thumb is one hour of research max per day for a healthy balance. Or thirty minutes and spend that other thirty minutes taking a long, hot bath!

Keep Track of Everything

Part of becoming an expert in your child's treatment and getting your shit together is organization. You want to come to appointments ready to ask questions and have a full understanding of what your child is taking, potential reactions, and contraindications. As I mentioned in the last chapter, it's ideal to have another person with you at appointments, or during morning rounds, as sometimes it's a lot to process what's being said and take notes. Or, if you are solo, voice record the meeting on your phone.

There are many ways to keep track of your child's treatment plan, so ask your oncology team what's the simplest way to provide you with an ongoing list of current meds and potential side effects.

> ### 💡 Toolbox Tip:
>
> A treasured friend of Cecilia's from college is an AML/BMT survivor and a med student. She rocks. She offers this sage advice: "Knowing the drugs your child received and the side effects they (could) cause can help with a variety of long-term treatments. My oncologist wrote up a ten-page document outlining all my chemotherapies, bone marrow transplant medications, side effects, and known future risks. It also included the annual or

semi-annual health screens I should receive (i.e., echo, EKG, DEXA scan, etc.). Every family member has this document saved, and I give it to every new doctor I see. This also takes the pressure off to remember everything during treatment. With technology advancing, another strategy could be to download the After Visit Summary notes from all the visits (usually on MyChart or a similar app) and save them to a folder." – Brooke Vittimberga, AML/BMT survivor and medical student

Talk It Out

While gaining knowledge is a huge part of getting your shit together right now, equally important is tending to your mental health. It's normal to be drenched in fear and panic right now—you are in animal instinct, mama-papa bear, fight-or-flight mode. You need to be able to express your fears to somebody, to cry or talk it out. But when you step back for a second and think about it, the last thing you want is for your baby to see your fear. Your child needs to feel powerful and kick-ass. Seeing their mom or dad cry because they are worried about them isn't terribly empowering.

Look for that support person or get your butt into therapy so you can regularly vent and restore your sanity. If you find yourself alone and feel that wave of fear and anxiety washing over you, find a nice place to hide from the kids and let it all out. Then wash up and greet your family with a hug and a smile. Our little red bathroom was my spot. Arne and I (unintentionally) rotated who was falling apart and while we often railed at each other, we found it wise to give each other a break and implode with a therapist or good friend instead, especially during these early, tender weeks.

♀ Toolbox Tip:

If you have a therapist, make an appointment right now (over Zoom so you don't have to leave the house or hospital), and if you don't have one, talk to the hospital social worker who can put you in touch with parent groups or someone to talk to who's been down a similar road. BetterHelp and Talkspace apps are fantastic for quickly securing an appointment with a therapist for your needs.

Following these action items and Toolbox Tips early in treatment will help you become calmer and more secure in the knowledge that, yes, you can do this. With this newfound knowledge and organization comes comfort for both you and your child and a greater sense of power over this seemingly powerless situation. You will take charge of what you can control vs spiraling in fear about what you can't control. With knowledge and organization comes comfort, for both you and your child, and an opportunity to let go of your fear—even for the briefest of moments—and find the joy and fun in life that still exists all around you. Now, let's get to creating that New Normal.

5

Establishing Your New Normal

Courage is not the absence of fear,
but the ability to act despite it.
ARCHBISHOP DESMOND TUTU

Cancer sucks for lots of reasons, not the least of which is the length of treatment. It sometimes feels endless and is endless, and that's without any relapse. When will life return to normal? With cancer, it's not like you simply get a diagnosis, kick the cancer's butt, and move on quickly. There's the long diagnosis and staging process, then treatment, and sometimes surgery and radiation. Even when treatment is done, there remain long months or years of follow-up care to make sure the cancer stays away.

Cecilia's diagnosis at age three involved a two-and-a-half-year marathon of treatment and years of follow-up. But establishing her new normal didn't stop at the end of treatment. In elementary school, high school, and college, she had strained conversations with her pediatrician and doctors she saw on campus when they learned about her cancer history. They were ill-equipped to answer any of her questions or concerns related to her childhood treatment. In her late twenties, Cecilia realized (and accepted) that being in her local Pediatric Survivorship Program was a smart choice. Instead of continuing with her regular doctor, who really didn't "get it", she now sees medical professionals who understand her past diagnosis and treatment, make wise suggestions about preventative testing, and see how bad-ass and powerful she is as a human. For the patient, redefining "normal" continues into adulthood as your child takes on ownership of their own well-being.

But right now, we are focusing on the present, and what's next for you, the caregiver. You've started to get your shit together in Chapter 4, and now establishing your new normal is the all-important next step. You and your family will probably be in cancer treatment and recovery for a long time, so finding ways to make it feel more normal is crucial for your day-to-day existence. You must normalize the abnormal to mentally and physically survive. Let me show you how.

Step One: Establish Boundaries

Once the initial shock and the first phase of treatment are behind you, you face forward and think, "Holy crap, how am I going to get to the finish line?" That's a big question.

For us, it started to click when we accepted our circumstances and surrendered to the reality of the situation at hand. We found that once we stopped rebelling against the diagnosis, we had the space to find our new normal by creating routines and boundaries that worked for us and our loved ones.

From years of observing interactions and conversations surrounding cancer, I have learned that it's paramount for patients and their caregivers to establish personal boundaries around the way they are treated with both words and actions in order to maintain some sense of agency and to lose the victim mentality.

Here's a great example from our experience mid-chemo: "She doesn't look sick" was an irritating phrase spoken far too often, in *front* of our daughter. Yes, cancer is scary, but usually, a child with leukemia (as well as many other forms of childhood cancer) is in clinical remission quickly since the initial phases of treatment knock the cancer down and subsequent years keep it that way. Therefore, a cancer patient is not sick, they are in *treatment*. That's more than simple semantics; it's a huge distinction from a mental health perspective.

It's up to *you* to make it clear to your medical team, family, and friends how you want them to talk about treatment at appointments, socially, and at school. Why? Because words matter. They can lift us up or destroy us in a second, especially when we are vulnerable. As an educator and mama of three, I've seen this happen countless times as children understand more than we realize. They will rise up or wilt under the seemingly innocent words and gestures of an adult.

💡 Toolbox Tip:

Empowering your child to feel strong, strong enough to fight this beast, strong enough to build up their ANC, strong enough to be the feisty kid who is going to fight, is your job. If they constantly hear "You're sick and weak", they'll start to believe it. Countless times at the hospital, we witnessed a child lose their power because of their own parents' fear and paralysis. Keep your language positive.

As you get past the flurry of a new diagnosis and settle into a routine, letting friends and family know what you need in terms of support and restating boundaries will be an ongoing conversation. For instance, they need to understand how serious it is if your child gets something as simple as a cold or fever on a playdate or at school. Before coming over to play, they need to let you know if they suspect any illness and keep their child home from school when sick. Finding a balance with your friends and family treating you as normally as possible while being as cautious as possible is a tall order. They will need guidance.

> **💡 Toolbox Tip:**
>
> Declare what you need in a friends-and-family email, on Facebook, or on CaringBridge.
>
> Every few months, we sent a detailed update with pictures and spelled out exactly what we needed from the people we loved. Friends and family love to help and to get guidance on what you actually need and want. Help them help you.
>
> *A full list of what to ask for and how to ask for it is in Chapter 6

Step Two: Normalize the Abnormal

It bears repeating: If your child's cancer treatment is lengthy, as they usually are, finding a way to make this new situation as normal as possible is essential for your mental and physical well-being as well as that of your entire family. We are not meant to live in fight-or-flight mode for sustained periods of time. Medication needs to be taken, shots endured, and a medical schedule must be followed. Making that as ho-hum as possible really helps your child shrug their shoulders and surrender into the routine versus fighting it. And if your child is happy, you are happy.

In order to establish your new routines, involve your child in the decision-making process and find a way to make it fun! Here's a story that might help you craft your own new normal.

At the end of Induction, our oncology nurse asked Cecilia if she wanted to come in for her weekly labs and chemo shots or have her parents learn to do them at home. "At HOME!" she said with a smile. Dear Lord . . . I think her nurse knew that being at home was probably the healthier option for Cecilia and nudged her toward that choice. You really can't say, "No, honey, I'm not down for that", but we sure wanted to for a hot second.

However, that nudge from our nurse sent us down an empowering path we could have never anticipated.

Bringing home a load of containers labeled biohazard and being trained to forcefully impale our child with chemo in her thigh was daunting. You can't give her a bit too much. Or too little! And her thigh has to be cold enough to numb the pain. And be sure nobody in the house—human or animal—touches the chemo. It was a lot to process. But slowly and surely, we got used to it and with Cecilia's input (crucial) created an awesome routine that included tacos and *Dragon Tales* with dinner and a sugar-free popsicle for dessert. Cecilia knew the shot had to happen before she could have the popsicle, so when she was ready, she would sit on my lap with the cold spray and ice pack, focus on Dragon Tales, count to three, and do her "whale breath" exhale as my husband Arne did the deed. Insert popsicle.

I swear to you, not a single tear was shed in all those years. Why? Because although we had boundaries, we gave her power. Donuts were not a dessert option, and whining was not permitted if she wanted to watch Dragon Tales with dinner. But she did get to pick the menu, watch a special show with dinner, and most importantly, she determined exactly how she wanted to get her shot. She created the rules, and the fun, surrounding that weekly, nasty methotrexate poke. In her eyes, the good far outweighed the bad.

💡 Toolbox Tip:

Maybe going to the hospital every week for a standard shot of chemo is good for you and stress-reducing! More time away from the hospital ended up being better for me. The key is to be in conversation with your child and intentionally create routines and rituals that serve you both. Take ownership of this process vs letting the situation own you by talking with your child now about what worries them, observing how they react in different medical situations, and then deciding what stresses you out the most. From there, you pick how you want to handle the basics.

Another idea to help normalize the abnormal is breathwork, which is a tried-and-true way to manage pain. Introduce your child to breathwork early so you can use it for routine things like bloodwork and other IV insertions.

> 💡 **Toolbox Tip:**
>
> Practice makes perfect. Before you go to your next poke, practice by having your child take a slow breath in for a count of three, hold it for two or three seconds, and then breathe out big (we called it Cecilia's "whale breath") as you lightly pinch their arm or otherwise gently simulate when the needle happens. Once it's done, have them take another deep inhale/exhale. The American Institute of Stress says deep breathing gives your brain a boost of oxygen and signals your parasympathetic nervous system to calm down, helping both you and your child feel a bit more Zen in the moment. Consider purchasing a child's doctor kit so they can practice on themselves.

There are other fantastic modalities for managing pain with breathwork or even self-hypnosis. You'll find links in Resources.

Step Three: Create Routines

Does your child have a weekly shot or nightly pill to take that they really hate? Involve them in the creation of traditions surrounding those dreaded daily pills and shots that simply have to happen and sprinkle in some joy along the way to normalize the process.

My favorite routine was the weekly lab. Rather than going to the hospital for labs like most of our peers, I decided to make it fun as well as less stressful and germy. I found a lab within biking distance and once a week I loaded Madi and Cecilia into the bike trailer with a pile of books and grabbed a much-needed workout around the neighborhood, ending up at the lab. Cecilia and our local phlebotomist got to know each other, and he respected Cecilia's request to be allowed to sit on Mama's lap as he slowly said, "One, two, three, GO!" and inserted the needle while her baby sister held her other hand. She never cried because, again, she had the power.

Afterward, we went out for bagels for a treat for the girls and a latte for me. Heaven. By the time we biked home, the lab results were waiting for me. Doing weekly labs this way relieved any anxiety Cecilia might have felt going to the hospital for labs and distracted me like crazy until I received her results and exhaled. She was still cancer-free.

New routines like this one must be created to help you through your journey and to empower your child to handle their daily treatment over the long haul. Shots are scary—even for adults! They look scary, they kinda hurt, and if we tense up it really is so much worse. And pills! Swallowing them can be hard for a child. With your child, identify what scares them the most and find ways to help them make that scary thing less daunting.

💡 Toolbox Tip:

If taking pills, or the taste of pills, stresses out your child, a stack of 6mp tablets fits perfectly into an empty gel cap that you can get at any pharmacy. These gel caps mask the bitterness and often can fit more than one pill—voila!

Be sure to check with your medical team, as many pill forms of chemotherapy also come in liquid form. Liquid or pill, some kids do well when you mix it into something else, such as a bit of unsweetened applesauce or a healthy smoothie (just be sure they finish the entire thing). See what works best for your child.

Parent hack: To help my two-year-old practice with pill swallowing, we started off practicing with mini M&Ms! He could practice swallowing small things (and get some chocolate candy while he was at it) and then worked his way up to bigger pills.
—JEAN, CANCER MAMA

Great advice! And mind the sugar. Make this a special circumstance.

The sooner your child finds tools and tricks to manage pain like Cecilia did, the sooner you can normalize these weekly procedures, removing the drama and tears from the situation. Use the tips and tricks above to give your child a sense of control. Fears and tantrums will be lessened, or—as was the case for us—eliminated altogether. Pick one idea and give it a try. You'll see how creating a sense of calm around your child's treatment will benefit you and your entire family's mental health.

Step Four: Creating A New Normal for Your Home

As your child starts cancer treatment and throughout the process, their ANC (absolute neutrophil count) is likely to stay low. This is a common side effect of treatment and means your child will be more prone to catching infections—something you definitely want to avoid. A simple cold or fever can land you back in the hospital for observation and may even delay their treatment.

One of the most effective ways to keep your child—and the rest of the family—healthy is to clean up your environment. Yes, I'm talking about your home. It's empowering to know that you can create a safe space, at least within your four walls.

Here's a list to get you started.

- Have everyone who enters your house remove their shoes before coming inside. Your shoes are the biggest germ tracker in your home and keeping germs outside—or at least just inside the front door—protects you and your child from outside germs.

- Establish a hand-washing routine: Insist that everyone in your family and anyone visiting hits the sink and washes up for thirty seconds with a generous amount of soap as soon as they arrive. Sing *Happy Birthday* once through slowly (no cheating), and you're done!

- As tempting as it is to bleach the crap out of everything, don't. Everyday cleaning products with ammonia or bleach are toxic and can be brutal on your child's immune system (seriously, Google this). Even worse, these environmental toxins put extra strain on the liver, which is already working overtime to process chemo.

A study, published in Chemosphere, analyzed thirty cleaning products, including multipurpose and glass cleaners, air fresheners and more. The study revealed that these everyday products may release hundreds of hazardous volatile organic compounds known as VOCs.

VOCs in cleaning products affect the quality of air both indoors and outdoors. But they contaminate indoor air two to five times more than outdoor air, with some estimates putting it as high as ten times more. Some products emit VOCs for days, weeks, or even months. "This study is a wake-up call for consumers, researchers, and regulators to be more aware of the potential risks associated with the numerous chemicals entering our indoor air," said Alexis Temkin, Ph.D., a senior toxicologist.

Sounds scary, right? So don't take any chances. Switch up your cleaning routine now by going "green," meaning ditch the products loaded with harmful chemicals. Use ones that clean just as well, smell great, and won't put your family at risk. It's a simple change that makes a big difference.

⚲ Toolbox Tip:

Green house-cleaning products (including laundry products) are commonly found at Target, large grocery stores, and online. More expensive does not mean better! Find what fits your budget and get cleaning. You can even DIY these products if you have the time.

Remember to look for non-toxic versions of any household items you buy, from furniture (which can off-gas for years) to carpets and paint. Finding non-toxic versions is easy.

See Resources for tips on making your house green forever.

Step Five: Creating Your Positude—Positive + Attitude

In chapter 1, I told you the story of how Cecilia invented the word Positude as her way of bringing a positive attitude to the daily crap she had to face during treatment. As you are now creating your new normal, this is a perfect time to look for ways to encourage your child, your family, and yourself to see the good things in your day so everyone can be fortified with positive images and words to better handle treatment. If your child is young enough, they likely won't realize the mortality issues surrounding their care, which is a blessing. Keep it that way by intentionally crafting your new way of life, boundaries, and routines with love and a positive vibe.

We were incredibly lucky to have a caregiver at the time of diagnosis named Joni. Joni is one of those smart, kind, and super intuitive people who connect with young children. Right after Cecilia's diagnosis, we watched Joni work her magic as she made Cecilia laugh, seamlessly steering her clear of germs and sneezes at the park and giving her the gift of play.

One day, during her pre-nap story time, Joni introduced the idea of an animal spirit to Cecilia. They had read about them in a book and Cecilia was mesmerized by the idea that we all have an animal spirit inside, protecting and defending us. Joni asked Cecilia what animal spirit was inside her, protecting her from cancer. "Dinosaurs!" she declared. Joni went on to guide Cecilia over the next weeks and months to define exactly which kinds of dinosaurs were killing different "bad cells" in her body and which were "on patrol."

The idea of applying a positive attitude towards life, and its impact on healing, is well-researched. Cecilia's dinosaurs were the beginning of our new normal, cementing our Positude, because they gave Cecilia the desire and power to fight by changing her mindset about her experience. Rather than seeing cancer with fear and herself as a victim, she was hell-bent on kicking cancer's butt because she had a way to control that part of her world through imagination and play. Friends and family slowly helped her build a toy menagerie of dinos. She visualized them fighting for her, acted that out through play as she repeatedly told the story of her dinosaurs destroying her cancer. She became one massively positive warrior. And thus, our new normal began.

> *The patients I've seen in practice who succeed (emotionally) all have a really good attitude. They were NOT victims. These are the cards they were dealt, and they go for it. Attitude. You gotta take care of that.*
> **—DAN LABRIOLA, ND**

6

Don't Be A Hero, You Already Are

Heroes don't have the need to be known as heroes, they just do what heroes do because it is right, and it must be done.

SHANNON A. THOMPSON

You never forget that wash of shock, fear, and utter paralysis when your doctor shares the news that your child has cancer.

As much as you want to crawl back under the blankets after getting that call, life in the childhood cancer world quickly demands that you wake up, pay close attention, and get organized as you become the unwitting advocate and gatekeeper for your child's treatment years and follow-up care. And nobody tells you this is what you've signed up for, at least not in the medical community—they are busy saving your child's life, after all.

As you have learned, after those first few days in the hospital for diagnosis and staging, it's time to go home and start living in this new normal. We are clearly expected to quickly get our shit together and do this on our own. I remember being told that Cecilia was "stable", and we could "manage" at home. I mentioned this story in Chapter One but let me really break down the drama for you and what happened next!

I distinctly remember the meeting with the nurse in the hallway outside of Cecilia's hospital room as she gave us our outpatient instructions. She handed over the list of chemo to get at the pharmacy, instructions for taking the meds (timing was crucial), reminded me of the seventeen times we had to come back to the hospital in the next month, and noted the long list of scary side effects while reminding us to stay vigilant of fever. I felt my eyes grow huge, and my mouth hung open in disbelief. At the end of her recital, she said brightly, "You've got this!" My copious tears said otherwise. GOT THIS? I wanted to bring that nurse home with us to be reassured of what to do next and to keep us from making a life-altering mistake. I felt the overwhelming need for help and had no clue how to ask for it or exactly what we needed help doing—aside from everything. And like many of you, I also had to figure out how to somehow take care of our other daughter, a dog, two cats, and my partner. Oh, and me.

Your child's cancer diagnosis is an unexpected and heroic call to action—and I'm fairly sure you didn't sign up to be a hero. I sure didn't. A few short months after her liberation from cancer, my incredible dad—one of our heroes and a constant support throughout treatment—was diagnosed with esophageal cancer, and I found myself bouncing from being the hero support for my daughter, to being the same for my dad. So, I know a thing or two about what it's like to be a caregiver to someone you love. The anxiety. The fear. The omnipresent grip of despair. You feel like you must do it all because you are their person, or because you think you have all the current data, or because you convince yourself that if you just try a little harder, you can fix them. People call you heroic or say, "I could never do what you're doing." I wanted to yell back at them, "Nobody gave me a CHOICE."

Sound familiar?

The Art of Not Doing it All Yourself

When I choose to see the positive things that came from our cancer experiences with my daughter and Dad, learning to ask for help is at the top of the list. Asking for help does not come naturally to most of us, even less so when you are under the intense stress of a new cancer diagnosis. How do you know what to ask for when you can't even form a sentence?

Over time, and with lots of trial and error, I learned that help comes in many forms and evolves as you find resources, develop trust with certain new and old friends, and, most importantly, figure out what you need. Because you already are a hero. And even heroes need support, a squad, back-up.

This chapter provides out-of-the box thinking about what to ask for and how to develop your own needs list and a support team to take some of the daily and weekly pressure off your family. Many of the following tactics that we used during treatment I also employed years later when a friend or family member had their own crisis. I can tell you from both the giving and receiving end, they work.

Note for those far from friends and family: Talk with your hospital social worker or the Child Life Services representative. Many hospitals have regular volunteers who are ready, trained, and willing to help you while inpatient, and often at home, too. Consider reaching out to your neighbors (even if you are new to the area). Let them know what's going on. You'll be surprised to see who shows up to help. As you read this next section, imagine help coming from these places.

Getting Started

When your child is diagnosed, it's important to remember that your friends and family are in shock too, so in the beginning, they may not be super helpful. Give them this book and direct them to Chapter 16, written especially to give them guidance to help support you!

Grandparents suffer; close friends and their children do as well. Sometimes their fear results in silence or a seeming absence from your life as they navigate their own feelings and process their own fears and "give you space." This can be hard to bear from people you love and who you thought loved you back.

Try to remember that the "C" word freaks everybody out and friends and family rarely get what you are going through. How could they? Instead of suffering in silence and frustration, empower them. Tell them what you need!

> 💡 **Toolbox Tip:**
>
> How to start? Assign one person you love and trust to be your Point Person and have them organize life for you. Have a meeting and really share with them what would be helpful so they can organize everything. Remember this—people LOVE a job and generally want to help. For easy access and updates, set up a Google Doc that itemizes what you need and when, and let a friend or family member send it out once or twice a week. Remember to add all those little errands that need to be done—pick up the dry cleaning, drop off a package, take your youngest to and from dance class, etc. Your Point Person can organize everything listed below.

I'll Tell You What I Want, What I Really, Really Want

Here is the list you've been waiting for! Use it, add your own special needs, and go for it:

Meal Prep

Have your Point Person assign one friend or a family member to set up your food requests on a site like mealtrain.com, where you can specify your family's wishes for meals and the appropriate days and times for delivery. Consider having dinner delivered for the first month or two of treatment as you get your bearings, and a couple of times a week thereafter.

💡 Toolbox Tip:
Set up a large cooler outside your front door for meal deliveries. You may want to chat, you may not, or you might be at the hospital. A cooler gives you options. Along with the cooler, put a sign over the doorbell that says, "nap time!" to preserve the quiet. You won't always feel like giving people an update and managing their emotions.

Weekly Groceries & Errands
Have your Point Person set up a Google Doc and send it out once or twice a week with your needs. Remember to add all those little errands that need to be done—pick up the dry cleaning, drop off a package, take the dog to the vet, etc.

💡 Toolbox Tip:
People will sometimes offer to pay for those groceries and errands. Let them and pay it forward later.

Updates
Everybody wants an update, and talking on the phone or sharing on social media might be great for you or be just way too much to handle during treatment, especially in the beginning weeks.

Have your Point Person recruit a friend, family member, or beloved teenager in the neighborhood to set up a webpage for your loved one's treatment with pictures and a general description of the current situation. Then, either you can go onto the site when you want to share news, or you can email or text your Point Person what you want posted.

💡 Toolbox Tip:
You can set up a site in a variety of ways, from creating a Facebook page to using the popular CaringBridge website at www.

caringbridge.org. This is an excellent space to also ask for what you need.

Help During Hospital Stays

Some hospital stays are a planned part of treatment, and others are a total surprise. Childhood leukemias can have up to six planned hospital stays for more intensive chemo that must be monitored more closely. And a fever will always mean a trip to the hospital for observation and possible intervention because your child's ANC is low, and they may need help fighting an infection. If your child is in-patient and stable, you will need some boredom relief while you endure your stay (see Chapter 9, The Hospital Party for ideas for planned stays!).

The Consolidation phase of treatment varies for different kinds of cancers. For ALL, it is normally right after a child is in remission and can involve hospital stays for intensive chemo. For us, it was six planned hospital stays. Visits from friends broke up our day beautifully when we were in the hospital. Depending on what you need, that visit might be a friend delivering your favorite coffee to you before she heads to work, dropping off dinner, or doing a puzzle with your child while you take an hour to walk outside and breathe. These small asks for help are lifesavers when you are enduring long days and potentially spending weeks in the hospital. Small asks add up to big help in the long run.

♀ Toolbox Tip:

Remember that your child needs a break from you, too. If allowed, have a favorite buddy come over to watch a movie or play together while you and their parent chat outside the room. If you are struggling, this can be a great way to find a private moment with a friend to decompress out of your child's sight. They don't need to see you cry.

Only invite those friends that you know will "bring the party" in terms of attitude and fun. It's not your job to help them feel better about your situation—you need them to lift you up! Surround yourself with people who bring a positive outlook to your hospital stays and encourage them to visit regularly or schedule time for a phone call or Facetime when you need a lift.

When we were in-patient and stable, our besties would make a point to come once a week with takeout and a game. We left that hospital room, dragging the IV pole of chemo with us, and had picnic dinners in a quiet, sunny public alcove.

Getting out of your room, when allowed, completely changes your mindset and offers some fun and normalcy to the day.

Help Just for You—The "Special Treat"

My parents taught me that it's the little things in life that really brighten your day. Fresh flowers in your kitchen from the garden, a lovely cup of tea, playing music you love, can change your outlook. During this marathon, what would be a special treat just for you?

What do you need help with, mentally and physically? Parents often forget to ask for help for themselves, but we need it! Our minds, bodies, and souls need regular tending so we can be the fierce advocate our child needs.

This is a very different ask for help than we have been discussing in this chapter. This ask for help isn't tactical; it's an ask for help that will give you space to breathe, reset, and recharge.

⚛ Toolbox Tip:

Friends at work or school love to band together to help. So let them help you. When you are making out your family's master list of needs, remember yourself. What would be helpful on a regular basis and bring you joy? Massages at home? Mani-pedi coupon? Free babysitting? A house cleaning service a few times a month? Put it on your list and ask boldly.

Thanks, But No Thanks

As important as it is to know what you need help with, it's equally important to know what you don't need. Well-intentioned people (and some not-so-well-intentioned folks) can really mess with your mojo if they come bearing gifts you don't want or stay longer than you can tolerate. So, grab some tea, find a cozy chair, and jot down your personal thanks-but-no-thanks list. I'll share my favorites below.

> ### 💡 Toolbox Tip:
>
> - Please don't refer to my child as "sick." Their cancer is in remission, they are "in treatment."
>
> - Please come to our home only when healthy. If you or a family member are sick, my child will get sicker and could end up in the hospital. Think COVID-19 restrictions.
>
> - When you come to our house, please take your shoes off by the door and wash up.
>
> - Never, ever say, 'I don't know how you do it." Neither do we. Instead, say, "You are doing an AMAZING job. Would you like a latte from Peets today?"
>
> - Never, ever say, "I couldn't do it (referring to a poke, hospital stay or cancer in general). And you think we can? Instead say: "You are a Warrior Goddess/God—I've got your back!"
>
> - Never, ever say; "God has a special plan for (fill-in-the-blank name)." God (or whomever/whatever you believe in), didn't create cancer and give it to my child. Or yours. God is hope and light and love.

A friend reminded me that I sent out an email early on about what not to do and say right after Cecilia was diagnosed and that it really helped our friend group immensely. See? Don't be afraid. Help people help you.

Cancer is scary. And sadly, it scares some people away when you need them the most. If you've done your best to be open to help, are specific about what you need and don't need, and a friend or family member is still MIA, then it might be time to part ways. You need your people to be there for you 100%, for better or worse.

That should get you started. If you remember nothing else from this chapter, please simply remember to say yes. Allow people to come into your life and take everybody up on any offer of help. You will be uplifted and stronger for the journey.

I want to remind you that Chapter 16 was written to help your friends, family, and parents understand all of this and more! Please share this book, and specifically that chapter, with them. If they are willing to read the entire book, all the better, because they will then fully understand what you are going through from a logistical and emotional standpoint without you having to spell it out.

Remember, you don't have to do it all to be a hero. You already are.

7

Advocating For
Your Child
"She'll Never Do Math or Science"

B y the time you read this chapter, I hope you've done some work finding that Hero Support from Chapter 6. Once you have that support in place, you can take action and learn how to advocate for your child.

From the minute Arne and I heard Cecilia had an eighty-five percent chance of surviving, we knew our job was to own the fifteen percent chance she had of dying. That fifteen percent was simply not acceptable—a roll of the dice. But how could we own it? What qualifications did we have to contribute to a positive outcome? As it turns out, a lot. And so do you, regardless of your child's specific diagnosis and survival rate.

The list of things you can learn about and advocate for is long and includes:

- Seeking options and advice for chemotherapy and radiation side effects. Every child is different, so start tracking your child's reactions now and share them with your oncology team.

- Learning about the power of eating well and how to make that part of your family's everyday life, even when your child does not feel well.

- Exploring complementary natural health therapies that work in conjunction with chemotherapy and radiation. This must be done with a professional in the field of complementary medicine in collaboration with your oncologist.

- Researching your child's protocol so you know your options.

- Learning the rules and regulations about hospital stays. You can advocate for lots of things, like the timing of a blood draw, or allowing your child to finish a nap before a procedure. Very often, the answer is, "Sure!"

To get you started, a full list of small and large things you can advocate for will be at the end of this chapter.

Knowledge of this new world you've found yourself in allows you to ask questions about options that can have critical short- and long-term implications for your child's health. Armed with that knowledge, you can advocate responsibly and fiercely for what's best for your kid and reduce your fear of the unknown.

> It's so easy to try to put your kid in a bubble because you're so fearful. I think the best thing to do is just to educate yourself on what truly is safe and not safe to do based on your child's actual protocol and not somebody else's. **—STACEY TEICHER, NP**

I realize that the concept of being your child's #1 advocate is intimidating. Heck, even this chapter title is intimidating. You might think, "I'm already slammed with this diagnosis, my family and work responsibilities and now I'm supposed to be the advocate for my child's deadly disease? No, thank you." I get that. Trust me, once you set up processes to get some help from friends and family for day-to-day operations, you can get this advocacy-ball rolling. You'll learn to use your resources and energy wisely (I'll show you how in Chapter 10) and see the positive outcomes in your child's long-term mental and physical health unfold before your eyes.

Being an advocate also gives you purpose and direction. Instead of spiraling in despair, fear, and constant what-ifs, you can engage with your medical team, actively contributing to decisions that can limit the effects of the drugs, which not only save your child's life but wreak havoc on their bodies and brains for years to come if you are not paying attention.

Pay attention.

The knowledge you will acquire as an advocate will help ease nagging fears that come with diagnosis. You'll have more facts at hand, know the right questions to ask, and won't sweat the small stuff.

Elevating Your Expertise

From the time your child is diagnosed, your education begins. And it's all overwhelming, especially at first as the language, the environment, and the entire situation feels alien and threatening.

♀ Toolbox Tip:

The strongest move you can make today is to take lots of notes on your laptop, phone, or audio recording device when your oncologist or nurse comes to see your child in-patient, or you have a regularly scheduled visit. Jot down your thoughts and concerns ahead of time and at the meeting so you can later reflect, do further research, and ask important questions the next time you see your medical team. Or email them right away if something seems off.

Your initial job as advocate is two-fold. First, learn the language of your child's cancer so you can communicate and contribute with your medical team effectively. And second, to become the #1 gatekeeper for your kid. Your medical team is amazing, and they are human. Mistakes happen, and your set of eyes on every situation, drug, lab draw, and test are a welcome and necessary part of the process. No one knows your child like you do. No one.

You can further learn to speak the same language as your oncologist by reading parent-friendly cancer sites, joining a Facebook group for your child's specific type of cancer, or reading up on protocol research websites. Parent groups can be the front line for quick information and reassurance when you are concerned about a reaction or curious about a drug. They do, however, tend to be intense and too emotionally charged for some. Strive to filter parental opinions from fact.

Pediatric cancer sites can give you pragmatic up-to-date research on drugs and statistics for your protocol that can be reassuring or terrifying, depending on what you are reading. Remember, your kid is your kid and not a cookie-cutter statistic, and their outcome and reactions are unique to them. The Resources section at the back of this book lists pediatric cancer parent sites and blogs, as well as information on how to find your child's protocol details. Dive in, take notes, and always question. That's how you become a kick-ass advocate.

💡 Toolbox Tip:

Take detailed notes to track how your child reacts to specific drugs. Use something that's easy for you: a Google Doc, journal, or phone notes app. Was drinking more water helpful? Were they nauseated when that was not expected? Then let your team know. We discovered through our online parent group that playing and sweating after a vincristine treatment could dramatically reduce the nausea and leg pains. We listened to those wise words and every time we had that drug, we surprised Cecilia with a sugar-free popsicle and a spontaneous trip to the park to run-run-run. She never had nausea or leg pain.

> One topic that is often overlooked is fertility—for all genders. Depending on the age of your child and the diagnosis, preventative action can be taken to preserve sperm and eggs. This isn't something you or your child are necessarily thinking about at this point, but it's important. Ask early, ask often, "Do we need to freeze, and can we do it now?"

Day three of treatment, our oncologist, who truly was and is wonderful, was going through the plan for our first month, which was called Induction. He reviewed Cecilia's statistics for survival, which is a tough thing for any parent to hear, and as we were leaving, casually said, "Oh, and by the way, she'll never do math or science. That's just something you'll have to accept as a side effect of treatment." I had zero knowledge at this point, and my only means of advocating for my child was to stare at him in utter disbelief.

Even at age three, our little girl was crazy about all things science, and she loved her numbers and books. My initial reaction was, "You're telling me she has a life-threatening disease that might take her from this world, and a cure will take away who she is inherently supposed to be? I don't think so." Mama Bear kicked in big time.

That conversation, and many others in the first months, was pivotal in forming the fortitude and awareness that I needed to take the reins on this terrifying situation. Gloom and doom forecasts for side effects, especially when highly successful interventions can change the course of those side effects, are not helpful. Constructive suggestions for alleviating side effects are what you need, along with a medical team that will listen when you tell them how your child responds to their specific drug cocktail.

Our oncologist didn't have the detailed research on hand about our protocol side effects, as he was busy putting her in remission and saving her life. Pointing us in the right direction to gain that information was my wish. We could have simply accepted what he said point blank, as many do. That blind acceptance, however, would have changed the course of Cecilia's outcome—and not in a good way.

Instead, I searched for the research team for her cancer protocol (POG 9201) and contacted them directly. Bold, right? I'm telling you, that's what happens when Mama/Papa Bear kicks in and you realize advocacy is up to you and you can make a difference. After the research director got over the fact that a parent was calling, he was incredibly generous, valuable, and kind. With his help, I discovered tactics and tips for Cecilia that allowed her brain to rewire itself, recreating neural connections that the chemo destroyed as it saved her life.

> ### 💡 Toolbox Tip:
>
> Formulate the questions and concerns you have regarding long-term effects as well as general questions about your child's protocol. Then, Google or ask your clinic for the names of the researchers on your child's protocol. Finding their contact information is easy and, in my experience, they are happy to take a call from a parent who has done their research. While many protocols now offer information on statistics online (not available when we were in treatment), it's still not enough. Call. Or you might get lucky and another parent may have done the work for you, so be sure to connect with a Facebook group for your child's cancer, if one exists. I suggest starting with your oncologist.

That lead researcher offered critical guidance for rewiring Cecilia's brain with games and activities that we could easily incorporate into her day—and we were able to easily make a fun part of her day. What your child may benefit from is unique to their diagnosis and protocol, but for us that included:

- memorizing basic addition, subtraction, and multiplication to fifteen
- math and logic games (Reader Rabbit was Cecilia's jam)
- gymnastics for balance and to alleviate neuropathy (mission accomplished!)

By the way, Cecilia graduated from Stanford University.

Undergrad and grad school, thank you very much. And she did lots of math and science while she was there, ultimately getting a master's degree in Community Health and Prevention Research from the Stanford School of Medicine, right next door to where she was treated as a little girl. Ironically and beautifully, her oncologist was a guest speaker for a Relay for Life event that Cecilia organized on campus with him. And yes, he was chagrined by his cavalier comment so many years before and so proud of his former patient and the beautiful life he helped save.

Barking Up The Right Tree—What Can You Advocate For?

There truly isn't an area where you can't advocate for your child. Sometimes, people get concerned that they will offend others or draw attention to themselves. Focus instead on your family. Think of all the little and big ways you can help treatment go smoothly and deliver these requests with firm kindness and love. If someone gets offended, they are not worth your time right now.

Here's a list of the many popular options for advocacy in the childhood cancer world, big and small, for you to choose from and add on to:

The Little Stuff

- How a lab is drawn: Which arm, your child on your lap or not, counting to three, etc.

- In-patient exams and labs: Don't wake up your child from a nap unless it's urgent.

- Social life: Create a system with friends for safely gathering, either in person, or schedule regular Zoom play dates so your child can keep up to date with their friends, no matter what.

- Hand washing and sanitizing: Required for anyone visiting your house or playdates.

- Home health: No shoes in the house (less germs!), healthy food options that are fun.

- Junk food limits: When people bring something over, request that no one brings cake, donuts, or excessive junk food.

> ### 💡 Toolbox Tip:
>
> Making a request like any of the above to nurses, a phlebotomist, friends, is best done before the event.
>
> Before you start a blood draw, tell your person, "Jack prefers the needle in his right arm after a count to four. Thank you!" Or when you arrive for an in-patient visit, make friends with the head nurse, and let them know you will put a sign on the door whenever your child is napping. Request that they reschedule any non-urgent visits or wellness checks. Kindness goes a long way when you make these kinds of requests—especially in the hospital or lab.

The Big Stuff

- What people have permission to say/not say: Your child is "in treatment" versus "sick", for example.

- Creating a new family food plan: Allow for fun, but take out unhealthy options. You are fighting a big fight—fuel yourself wisely.

- Protocol options: Can her labs be done at our neighborhood lab to avoid the hospital?

- Complementary medicine: What forms of complementary medicine will help your child's chemo work better? Ask if you can add an anti-nausea medication, or peppermint for your vomiting child, even though the data says it's not needed.

- Returning to school: Meeting with your principal and determining how concessions will be made for learning while on treatment, and how the school will make sure the community is asked to stay home when sick.

- Now is the time to advocate for your financial options. Reach out to your social worker to ask what kind of financial aid is available at the hospital or through various cancer organizations such as the Leukemia and Lymphoma Society. Your hospital social worker may also have assistance available, such as parking passes or discounts at the hospital cafeteria for longer stays. See Resources for examples of other organizations that may provide additional support.

💡 Toolbox Tip:

It's incredible what happens when you just ask. If your oncologist does not know anything about complementary medicine, connect with a practitioner who works in a hospital setting and set up a Zoom meeting. Sometimes, they are not in your area. We worked with Dr. Dan Labriola at Northwest Natural Health in Seattle.

Oncologists are specialists in their craft and normally will simply give a hard "no" to any form of vitamins or alternative care such as massage—and with good reason. Vitamin B9, or folic acid, is closely related to leucovorin, for example, and turns off the effectiveness of the drug methotrexate! But other vitamins and body care elevate the treatment and recovery. It took three months of nudging our oncologist before he would even speak to Dr. Labriola (and Dr. Labriola wouldn't work with us unless it was alongside Cecilia's oncologist—that's important).

A beautiful, respectful relationship was ultimately formed, as well as an awesome plan for helping Cecilia safely be her best on treatment. More in Chapter 11.

If nothing else, I hope this chapter empowers you to see the myriad ways you can, and should, advocate for your child. Nothing is off limits, so if something is important to you or your kid and not noted above, go for it! Remember, never forget that nobody knows your child like you do. Armed with growing knowledge, love, and compassion, you are ready to start advocating for your child today.

8

Hospital Stays

I'm gonna miss this place!

CECILIA, AGE 4

Treatment for many kinds of childhood cancers may include a Consolidation phase when chemotherapy is given to prevent cancer cells from coming back. Consolidation begins once your child goes into remission at the completion of the Induction phase. Protocols may have changed, but our protocol at the time required a series of six inpatient chemo treatments. Those usually last a minimum of three days, depending on how well a patient's liver processes the chemo. It's long. It's nasty. And if it goes well, super boring. Today, scheduled inpatient stays—depending on the diagnosis—can be much shorter. But remember, if your child gets a cold or fever they may be admitted for an extended time while they recover. Also, super boring.

Seeing that huge yellow IV bag labeled "biohazard" as Arne and I walked into Cecilia's hospital room for the first treatment was terrifying. But we made it, and on the very last day of five months of Consolidation, we finally rolled Cecilia and all our gear out of the hospital in her little red wagon. Arne and I looked at each other, noticing the huge bags under our eyes, and silently mouthed, "OMG, we made it!"

Meanwhile, Cecilia (fully aware that this was her last scheduled in-patient) wandered off to the front of the hospital, spun around slowly, and declared wistfully, "I'm gonna miss this place." Hearing this, we knew we had done something right.

Crafting Your Hospital Stay

Early on, as I looked over the entire treatment schedule and processed the enormity of this particular phase, I am not gonna lie, I felt a whole lot of fear and despair. I agonized about changing our secure routine at home, leaving my baby behind, potentially missing weeks of work, and stepping into a deeper layer of cancer-world that I didn't understand and was not ready to embrace. My head was full of all the things I'd heard in my online support group about everything that could go wrong during a hospital stay and I worried:

Could she handle the huge doses of chemo?

Would she be throwing up 24/7 and lethargic?

Could I sleep in the hospital?

What would we do all day?

How would Arne and I handle missing Madi and Madi missing us?

And how could I be sure she'd get out on time after three days?

Many cancer protocols stipulate that after chemo is administered, a patient's liver or kidney numbers must return to a level that indicates they are processing toxins out of their body and avoiding damage to other organs and the brain. They say this casually, but it's enough to make a parent freak out. I know I did. The focus becomes solely on those liver or kidney numbers because that's your ticket to going home and not having a train wreck. Kids can get out after three days, but often it takes days longer if their liver or kidney isn't happy. That's a lot of unknown for both parents and kids to process.

By the way, we always got out in three days. I'll give you my tips for that in Chapter 11.

While hospital stays are inevitable, they don't have to be filled with doomsday moodiness. Will you be bored? Probably. Will you sleep well? Probably not. Will you worry? That depends. You can bring a positive outlook to the inevitable hospital stay and I will show you how in this chapter with checklists for your stay and Toolbox Tips focusing on strategies for advocating for your child while they are in-patient. In the next chapter, I'll teach you how to bring your own party to these hospital trips to relieve stress and boredom, and to elevate serotonin.

As you may know by now, sometimes you'll have a heads-up when a hospital stay is approaching because it's a scheduled part of treatment. At other times, you may be admitted in a hurry for a fever or exposure to something such as chicken pox, which in our case arrived compliments of Cecilia's preschool bestie. While it's nice to thoughtfully pack for planned visits, it's also important to have a go-bag ready for unexpected trips to the hospital. It's natural to think about what your child wants and needs first, but I'm going to encourage you to think of your needs, too. That's why your go-bag items are noted first below. Use this go-bag list for your planned and unplanned hospital stays.

What's a go-bag? A go-bag is simply a list of creature comforts to bring from home to make sure both your child and you are more comfortable, more relaxed, and more at ease during your lengthy stay. Some stays are short, some are long, and all benefit from planning, when feasible.

When planning your child's go-bag, decide what would make your child happy and let them, within reason, bring it to the hospital. Include them in the creation of the go-bag list. This can be an empowering way to give them a little sense of control over their situation.

When planning your own go-bag items, think about those little things that will help you be a better person and give you strength. That might be your favorite tea, crossword puzzles, or movie downloads for your child's naptime. I strongly suggest bringing your own pillow and snacks.

Take a picture of this list and keep it handy or create your own list and tape it to the fridge. This glorious list is part mine, and it includes awesome ideas from my Facebook friends.

Your Go-Bag List:

- computer and charger for work and fun
- phone and charger
- portable charger
- extension cord*
- AirPods*
- preferred snacks*
- purse/ID/wallet
- medications and vitamins*
- busy work (book, sewing, etc.)*
- blanket, mattress topper, pillows (yours and your kid's)
- tennis shoes and slippers
- toiletries:*
    - toothbrush & toothpaste
    - deodorant
    - hair ties
    - shampoo/conditioner
    - brush

- body and face wash
- toilet paper (soft!)
- underwear
- hair dryer
- hand sanitizer or wipes★
- sleep mask★ or blackout curtains
- nice hand lotion★
- heating pad or warmie★
- lavender essential oil
- peppermint essential oil (for nausea)
- Tylenol★
- body and face towels
- nail clippers and file★
- three full outfits (more can be delivered later) including undies, plus cardigan or sweatshirt★
- coffee cup★
- water bottle★
- loose leaf tea and strainer so you can have your favorite tea★
- electric kettle★
- backpack or small bag for in-hospital travels★
- favorite candy★
- fan
- neck pillow
- robe
- earplugs★
- dirty clothes bag
- framed picture of family or friends

> 💡 **Toolbox Tip:**
>
> This is a list for both you and your child when you have the time to plan. For your emergency go-bag, consider having a second bag ready with just the items noted with asterisks (*). Keep that bag by your front door. If you have more lead time before a hospitalization, take your time packing but refer to your list so you don't have to second-guess yourself.
>
> For the lavender and peppermint tinctures, consider buying an inexpensive diffuser to run 24/7.

Strategies For A Healthy Hospital Stay

The Power of the Well-Placed Bribe

During a hospital stay, it's tempting to compensate for your fear and to make your child feel better by showering them with stuff, especially in the early days when everything is so new and scary. However, cancer-life will quickly become routine for your child if you help them see it as part of life, their new normal.

Overindulging your child gives them a reason to be a little tyrant (I knew a few) as children will cry at the drop of a hat if they realize they will be rewarded for any and all behaviors because their parents are scared. Our nurse practitioner, Stacey Teicher, is an incredibly gifted professional and she is magical with children. She kept the mood positive, even when preparing to do a lumbar puncture. She has observed that "So many children kind of became little spoiled brats because their parents felt so bad for them. They were given whatever they wanted, and this created behaviors that were unpleasant. If you are going to be in this for two and a half years, you don't want to create a child that is put on a pedestal. You want your child to still be able to take care of themselves and learn and thrive as normally as possible."

Wise words. There will be plenty of times when real tears are warranted, and you will learn to tell the difference quickly.

Conversely, rewards can be a powerful motivator for all the crap cancer kids must endure. Used in this way, a reward system (what I call the well-placed bribe) can be an incredibly powerful parenting tool.

Before you consider a reward system, think through how you communicate poke-and-procedure details with your child right now. Most of us avoid the conversation. Not only do we not want to talk about it, but we worry about what our child might do when they hear what's next. Cry? Throw a tantrum? Disrupt a moment of family peace?

But I can tell you from thirty years of experience as an educator and having gone down this childhood cancer road myself, that kids really don't like surprises, especially when they are sharp and painful. I learned from our family cancer therapist that talking through the steps over and over in the days leading up to a poke or procedure in a super matter-of-fact way could be remarkably effective in reducing Cecilia's fear and anxiety. That proved true.

Why?

Because the event was no longer an "unknown" and it became routine when she could repeat the plan back to us in her own words. Powerful. She grew to trust that we would never shock or surprise her with an invasive treatment, simply because we didn't want to talk about it ahead of time. And believe me, we really didn't. But remember, it's our job to be our child's advocate—even if that means we have to push back on our own insecurities and nerves.

Toolbox Tip:

"Play Procedure" is a real thing. Consider buying your child a doctor's kit and/or asking your medical team if you can take home supplies that look like a needle or bandage. If you're lucky, your nurse practitioner will loan you her stethoscope (our Stacey did!). Cecilia loved playing doctor on her stuffies. Often before a procedure, we'd find her acting out the details of her next poke and test … usually on her willing little sister!

After telling your child about the next event, establish a simple reward system so your child knows what is expected of them (being polite and kind, not throwing a tantrum) and what's going to happen (labs and an X-ray, for example).

> ### 💡 Toolbox Tip:
>
> Be mindful not to reward everything. We did in the beginning and quickly realized we would deplete our checking account if she got a Beanie Baby for every poke and procedure. It will be clear quickly what your child hates the most. Each child is different. Some might be fine with lab tests but refuse to eat anything but french fries. Choose your well-placed bribe wisely and remember, cancer is a marathon. Pace yourself and make your system sustainable.

One of the gifts of this journey is that your child can learn to build up their resilience, which is a beautiful thing in the long run. Once Cecilia learned how to "whale breathe" through her labs and IV insertions, she didn't need to be rewarded anymore and the strength she developed served her well during bigger treatments. We kept some no-sugar fruit seltzers on hand (she thought they were sodas) to help the oral medications go down and for processing higher doses of chemotherapy (more below). Sugar-free lollipops, popsicles, or a few gummies are always a great bribe for the smaller stuff.

> ### 💡 Toolbox Tip:
>
> It's common for children to lose their appetite because they simply don't feel well and feel nausea with some chemo. They protest their normal, healthy foods and stop eating or slow down their food intake. This can be triggering for many parents, who often resort to allowing their child to eat all forms of junk food just to get some calories. But remember, this marathon requires a strong body and soul. Don't bribe your child with sugary treats that will jack them up and make them crash in a few hours, doing nothing for their stamina or mood. Stick to healthy eating habits, lots of water, and avoid bribing them with junk food—it won't serve you or your child.

Creating Space

Once your child is in-patient, it's time to unpack your go-bag and settle in. Strive to make the space as cute and cozy as a hospital room can be and add all the little touches right away, such as family photos and pillows, so your child can see them and feel more secure.

Now it's time to connect with your nurse. Confirm the schedule that you discussed with your oncologist pre-stay and discuss options for your child that work best for their needs. For example, maybe your child is super excited to attend the hospital preschool, so ask that essential tests are done before or after preschool hours.

Remember, you know how to advocate for your child. Now is the time to make friends with your hospital team and make requests like these:

- Please do routine check-ups and pokes before or after nap time only.

- Middle-of-the-night vitals must be done with a flashlight. Please don't turn on florescent overhead lights, so my child can continue to sleep.

- If my child is well, we will take our chemo "on the road." Please facilitate us going to the playroom, to roam the halls, or to eat lunch outside.

- Please allow my child to pick where the IV will be placed. (IVs, especially in the hand, can be painful so don't allow anyone to put them in your child's dominant hand, and request that IVs are well-bandaged, so your child does not dislodge the catheter when they move around. Your child may prefer the IV in the crease of their elbow!)

- Allow your child to request the color of the Band-Aid or wrap after a lab or IV.

- If multiple sticks need to happen in one day (labs, IVs, tests, etc.) make sure they happen at the same time. Get them all over with at once and move on with your day instead of waiting around in anticipation for each one to happen.

- If your child is nauseous, ask for relief, even if it's not indicated as a side effect.

> A lot of the hospitals now carry peppermint and encourage you to put it on a cotton ball or they will bring one in to help with nausea. We ran a diffuser 24/7 and the nurses/staff all embraced it and called our room the happy Zen room with the fun smells.
> **—JILL, CANCER MAMA OF TEN-YEAR-OLD CANCER PATIENT**

Many hospitals have a toy box that they use as a reward for larger treatments, such as a spinal tap or bone marrow aspirate. Inquire if one exists (out of earshot from your kid), and make sure before the big event that there is something in there your child will love.

These procedures can be done under sedation (ask!), but they are still a big deal and worthy of a prize, sedated or not.

💡 Toolbox Tip:

Surprises happen and you'll need your calm advocacy skills to do what's best for your child. If a nurse comes in unexpectantly to do a lab or run a test, talk to them outside the room and explain that your child does best when informed ahead of time. Then, plan to do the poke or test after you've updated your child.

Sometimes the person who needs to run the test or poke your child can help you explain what's coming, as many have wonderful ways of engaging with children. But take it slow, and advocate for your kid—nobody needs to be in a hurry unless it's an emergency and you can lose your child's trust, and their trust for the medical team, if you throw unexpected pokes and tests at them regularly. Then, if a true emergency happens, you've built up a reserve of trust to get you through that experience.

If you don't have a "whale breathing" system in place for pokes like we did, contact Child Life Services at your hospital. With advance notice, they can send someone to help your child endure the IV insertion or lab. They might bring a squishy ball or other distracting device and may be able to coach your child on how to handle their pokes with less stress.

"Let Me Outta Here"

For many radiation and chemo protocols, there are benchmarks that a child has to hit to be released from the hospital. Talk with your oncologist before admission to understand what those are, and how you can help your child reach those goals. Bring your notebook and ask questions, do some research on your own, talk to parents who've "been there" and ask what tips they have for your stay and getting out of the hospital in a timely manner.

💡 Toolbox Tip:

Following up with your team with more questions as you prepare for a hospital stay is key. Your medical team expects you to know the timing of various drugs and if your child needs to be NPO (nothing by mouth) or have food on board for blood test or chemo day.

At our first hospital stay during consolidation, we witnessed our roomie Rebecca's parents in shock when they realized her four pm chemo had been missed and was time sensitive. This was a shock to us as well as, until then, we thought we had no role in administering her medication at the hospital. Wrong. Nurses are human. Have your pre-meeting, research, ask questions, ask more when you arrive, and check in with your child's nurse. Check again at every shift change.

There are two standard ways to metabolize chemo and get out of the hospital—movement and hydration. Both help flush out what is no longer needed after the medicine does its job. While it's tempting to stay in bed at the hospital and watch movies, get your child up and moving as much as they can by taking trips to the hospital library, playroom, cruising the halls with their IV poll, and even getting a bit of sunshine outside. All of this helps metabolize drugs and ease the muscle and joint pain that some drugs cause.

Hydration is key in flushing out chemo and radiation, so keep the sugar-free fluids going. I flavored Cecilia's water with some lemon or lime for fun. Keep your liquid choice sugar-free; cancer cells thrive off sugar. Sugar does not cause cancer. But cancer loves to feed off high sugar, high carb foods.

> 💡 **Toolbox Tip:**
>
> Have your child drink water before chemo and radiation. Drink water during chemo and radiation. Drink water after chemo and radiation. Not only does hydration help to process treatments, but it can also be important when starting a chemo round. Drugs, like methotrexate, require that a child's pH levels be at a certain point to even begin treatment. And your child needs to be well hydrated enough to dilute the chemo in their urine. Start that hydration push a full day ahead of your stay. This speeds discharge from the hospital by getting liver levels back to normal after an infusion. It also helps the liver process that wonderful, but toxic, stuff. Allowing your child to pick a cute reusable container helps with their buy-in! And make it a game! If they don't like to drink much, this is a great place for a well-placed bribe.

Before being admitted, refer to your pre-hospital stay notes and understand exactly what new drugs your child will receive. Then do your research and find the best way to help the drugs do their job and then get out of their system.

Vincristine is a powerful drug that can cause debilitating joint pain. When I read that Cecilia was going to be on it during her hospital stays, I did a little research and talked to my online cancer friends. I learned early on that a little sweat and movement helps ease pain tremendously if it's done before the pain sets in. I always planned a park or biking day after Vincristine because Cecilia loved it. This worked every time.

💡 Toolbox Tip:

Make movement fun and don't tell your child why you're doing it. What does your child love? A little baseball? A trip to the roller rink? Plan it. If you just offer up Disney channel and popcorn, they will go home and feel more miserable as the chemo will have a much harder time metabolizing when they are immobile.

Armed with your pre-stay meeting notes, go-bag for you and your child, strategies for a well-placed-bribe, and techniques for getting home more quickly, you are ready and, hopefully, empowered for your first stay! Remember that advocacy in the hospital is key, and this can be best done from a place of calm and kindness when at all possible.

Ready to bring on the party?

9

The Hospital Party

Celebration is my attitude, unconditional to what life brings.

RAJNEESH

As we approached our initial in-patient hospital stay, we made a choice and a decision—we surrendered and accepted this next phase of six planned hospitalizations and intentionally planned the details of our days like we were going to battle—very serious and more than a little grim. Then it occurred to us: We could stop worrying about the "what ifs" and just make it fun as Dr. Dahl suggests. Yes. FUN!

Enter the Hospital Party.

In anticipation of this part of treatment, I started hoarding all the little gifts people were showering on our family and collected inexpensive activities that I thought might be fun for a small child in confinement with an IV 24/7. Next, we bought bright, colorful room decorations at the Dollar Store to make the space more festive for Cecilia, us, and any roomie. We set up a routine with our parents to visit regularly, as they blessedly lived nearby, and made a giant, lively, poster board with the full schedule for each day.

We were ready.

You could hear my dad down the hall before you saw him. His big, Santa-Claus-style voice bellowing "Hello!" and "How are you doing?" to everybody he saw on the way to our room, stopping at the nurse's station for a quick "Did ya hear the one about?" joke.

My parents, Pauline and Glenn, made a point of arriving with bags full of fun, hearts full of love, and an abundance of positive energy. After a few weeks in cancer-land, they knew better than to shower us with concerned looks and tearful hugs. We needed (and asked for) Positude. Distraction. And for them to walk through that hospital door and take over. We gave them their notes for the day and then exited stage right as they took center stage, capturing their granddaughter's attention and giving us a break.

Dad was the Happiness Captain (and my inspiration), lifting our spirits with his big jovial voice and tons of yummy, healthy, "snicky-snacks." He could be counted on to pick up some decadent KFC just for fun, or swing by the farmer's market for an approved treat for Cecilia. Fresh fruit and quality protein from the farmer's market always did the trick, because finding healthy food in a hospital is not always easy. And he always included a joke gift, like the giant All detergent box he brought during one hospital party, filled with fresh flowers. "All" because Cecilia was kicking her **A**cute **L**ymphoblastic **L**eukemia's ass, and we'd just learned her blood type was A-positive. Based on those facts, Dad declared that Cecilia was going to be ALL right. All the signs were there. Get it? Find the "dad" friend or family member in your life and invite them to the party. They're the special person who brings lightness, joy, and fun to the day.

Mom distributed her carefully planned treasures during each visit to help keep Cecilia entertained. Cecilia's eyes would get wide as she spotted Grandma. She'd peek around her back for a hidden goodie. My mom never brought anything extravagant (be careful not to go down that road, or you'll get stuck), instead bringing something new to look at—a sticker book, or a new treasure you know they really want. For Cecilia, if it was a particularly big procedure day, it was a Beanie Baby!

Mom always made sure that she thought of me and Arne first with a surprise tea delivery or something cozy from home. I'll never forget the day I complained about how cold I was in the hospital. Mom showed up with my favorite Peet's sugar-free vanilla latte and a bag from the mall with a cozy new sweatshirt and pants. I felt so spoiled and will never forget that small, thoughtful kindness. Discover your "mom" and invite her to the party. That person is the cozy one, the thoughtful one who always thinks above and beyond, seeing exactly what you need before you even know it.

Arne's parents, Marie and Nils, took up the caregiving at home, tending lovingly to Madi and our pets in a way that touched us deeply. Marie formerly was a professional nanny and was the perfect choice to take on the details with Madi's care; she attentively maintained her schedule to the letter. Nils took up taking care of Max, our dog, and Tane, our kitty, and processed his fears and worries by fixing every little broken knob or loose screw in the house. They brought Madi with them to the hospital, visiting almost every day for a cuddle and visit with her "iss" (sis), to watch *Teletubbies* in bed (their special treat), or run down the hallways together giggling, Cecilia's IV pole flying behind them.

Marie and Nils were tactical in their help. Glenn knew how to bring a party. And Pauline was wonderful with errands and thoughtful treats. Our parents desperately needed something to do, something to defray the intense grief and fear they felt for us and their grandchild. Hospital parties became the perfect distraction. See Chapter 16 for more ideas specifically for grandparents and be sure they read this section of the book as well.

We were incredibly lucky to be close to our family, both literally and physically, and I know that's not always the case for a cancer family. If you are not close to your parents, find this kind of help in other friends and family who will show up for you. Use Pauline, Glenn, Marie, and Nils as examples of people using their gifts and talents for good and find and pinpoint those people in your life if you can.

> 💡 **Toolbox Tip:**
>
> Everyone needs a purpose on the team. You're the coach, calling the plays. As you figure out the best way for family or friends to help you during hospital stays, play to people's strengths, as we did with our family. This gives them purpose and helped us enormously because we knew our family was being emotionally and logistically lifted up with care at home and in the hospital.

So how do you create your own hospital party? It starts with a calendar.

Calendar Time

Before your first in-patient stay after diagnosis, introduce yourself to the people in charge of the children's hospital's fun. Typically, this department is called something like Child Life Services. It's their job to organize the playrooms, preschool, activities in the room if you are unable to leave, and outside activities if you are allowed to get some fresh air. A visit to the playroom or library can be a great time-killer and change of scenery. Explore what's available, along with all the time and location details, so you can plug that into your master calendar.

When a hospital visit is planned, making a daily schedule is a helpful way to create a sense of normalcy and to take away the fear of the unknown for everybody. As tempting as it was to stay in our sweatpants for our two-and-a-half years of treatment, we got up and got dressed, even in the hospital. Once Cecilia laid out cute clothes to pack and her favorite stuffed animals and pillow, she was good to go for our stay.

We made our master schedule on a poster board and color coded the time and activities from Child Life Services, trips to the playroom, cafeteria, library, visits from friends, interspersed with pokes and procedures. That way, she always knew what was coming while still having something to look forward to or focus on instead of just waiting for the inevitable fearful parts of the day. Cecilia helped plan and decorate the board with markers and stickers so she was fully invested in the process. Here's a classic schedule template that we used successfully for years.

Schedule Template

7:00 am	Rise and shine! (Rounds by the doctors began typically at 7am)
7:00–9:00 am	Breakfast, lots of water
	Text Grandma and Grandpa for lunch request. Labs in IV, nurse check (no new pokes!)
	Get dressed for _____
9:00–10:00 am	Preschool! (This is typically an hour off for us.) Bring your water bottle.
10:00–11:30 am	Quiet playtime in our room. Window cling-art.
11:30 am	Refill your water bottle!
	Text Tracy and Stuart dinner request
11:30–2:00 pm	Grandma and Grandpa lunch and playtime!
2:00–3:30 pm	Rest time. Nap or reading time only.
3:30–4:00 pm	Playroom visit!
4:00–5:30 pm	Scan with nurse Leslie, then a MOVIE!
5:30–7:00 pm	Tracy, Stuart, and Grace visit
	Eat takeout in the lobby and play Go Fish
7:00–8:00 pm	TV time
8:00–8:30 pm	Into jammies, warm milk, and massage. Wave music on.
8:30 pm	Lights out

You may have hours, days, or weeks with your child as an in-patient. Once you know the potential length of your stay, strive to make your schedule before your trip, if it's a non-emergency stay, or you and your child can create it together once you've arrived and are settled in if you land in the hospital unexpectedly. If you'd rather not make a schedule yourself, text your Point Person with the activities and times, the people you want to visit, requests for food or coffee, etc. Allow that person to make your daily chart for you and your family.

Now What?

Okay, you made it! Your child is now in-patient. The room looks cute. You've got your go-bag unpacked, you've scheduled visits from your family or friends and set up a plan for activities with Child Life Services.

All of that is amazing. But you still have a lot of hours to kill in a tiny room, and watching videos all day isn't good for anyone. What are you going to do to avoid losing your sanity? Check out the Resources section at the back of this book for a list of top toys and activities for kids (and parents) who are stuck in a small room for hours on end. They are fun, creative, and really help to pass the time. Best of all, they are tried and true, so there is no guesswork for you.

As you review the Resources section and create your own activity and toy shopping list, be sure to encourage pretend play. A box of toy animals, Felt Kids, Legos, and art projects allows kids to come up with their own storyline instead of following a prescribed narrative. This helps kids in trauma process their feelings in a healthy way. One clever parent shared with me that when her daughter was being particularly steroid-driven, she would make her own "emotions" game.

> I would make faces of each emotion and let her name it, then discuss how she is feeling now. Sometimes I use this when she has a tantrum. For example, if she is feeling mad, we take deep

breaths and discuss if she needs time to think. It's not always pretty or easy, but it helps her recognize emotions. If she is sad or nervous, we talk about it and discuss ways to cope. If she is happy, we dance/ do something silly and embrace those moments.
—ANONYMOUS

💡 Toolbox Tip:
When picking things to do, keep in mind that your child will probably be hooked into an IV via a port, or in their arm or hand if there isn't a port. Look for activities that won't hurt or can be done one-handed. Remind the staff to put the IV in your child's non-dominant hand if possible!

Share the Resources section with your Point Person so they can ask far-away friends and family to send stuff to you. Or ask a local friend to find items for you at the Dollar Store or shop online so your supply is ready to go. If people insist on paying, let them. You'll pay it forward in years to come. Save a few items for treats or rewards for after a major treatment, scan, radiation, or a particularly bad day.

Keep It Special
The key to a successful hospital party is novelty. When a child must face a few days or weeks of living at the hospital, having new things to look forward to really helps lighten their mood.

💡 Toolbox Tip:
After a hospital party, put all the rewards, treasures, books, toys, and decorations away and do not let them see the light of day until the next visit. That keeps them special and a beloved tradition, something to look forward to when your child must be admitted again.

Cecilia grew to love her afternoon "wanders" around the ward and never failed to drag her IV pole along and entertain the nurses' station with knock-knock jokes or bring a neighboring child a picture that she drew just for them. Laughter and kindness are good medicine. So is focusing on others. This goes for you as well. Once you are in the swing of treatment, keep an ear out for newly diagnosed parents who could use a cup of coffee and a compassionate and understanding ear.

Focus Outward

When you or your child feel a little blue, it's time to take a walk and see who else you can engage with on your floor, and who might need some cheer. Making gifts or art projects for other kids on the ward or for the nurses' station gives both you and your child something to do and someone else to focus on. That's good energy. If allowed, let your child deliver those cards, gifts, or art projects in person.

> ### 💡 Toolbox Tip:
> Nurses are a great resource for introducing your family to another child who might be able to play, or a newly diagnosed family needing moral support. Consider bringing an activity or game that can be shared since parents sometimes can't stay with their child all day due to work. Or let your child pick something from your hospital party stash and gift it to a new friend down the hall.

When Friends Visit

Breaking up your day with visits from friends and family is a fabulous distraction and can provide a sense of normalcy— if you pick the right people to visit. Make sure you plan around scheduled treatments, avoiding post-procedure times so your child can recover, and don't allow visits too close to rest time. Your child will need and want to feel fresh and ready for fun.

Some friends and family don't have the right mojo for your hospital parties. For example, if a girlfriend just won't get beyond the "C" word and can't bring the fun to her visit, ask her to help in another way. One good friend constantly said on repeat, "I could never do this. How do you do this every day? If this was my child, I would dissolve." Not helpful. Don't invite that friend back to your hospital parties. I didn't.

It's possible that your friends and their kids may be a little scared to visit the hospital. That's okay. Help them by sharing what they can expect and encourage them to talk about it ahead of time with their child (if they bring one). Then give them ideas about what they can bring to the hospital party.

What to Expect When You Visit Us at the Hospital:

- If anybody arrives with even the sniffles, the hospital won't let you in, so please stay home and get well soon! We'll miss you and see you later.

- There are often extensive check-in protocols and procedures, so plan on arriving an extra ten minutes ahead of time to get all of that done.

- Priyanka will have lots of wires and an IV attached to her hand.

- Christian might not be in a great mood, or be in a great mood, or both during your visit!

- There will be beeping from the monitors, which is constant and intimidating. Not to worry, they are just checking Alice's status.

- Hospitals smell weird—part cleaning products, part medicine, probably part poop!

- Hand sanitizer and hand washing stations are everywhere and need to be used all the time. Cancer kids are immune compromised, so they get colds and flu easily. Help us by keeping your hands clean all the time and keeping your child's hands clean as well.

- Bald heads are prevalent on our ward, which can make you sad, but it's the least of a cancer-parent's worries.

Please don't stare. Just smile and have fun with them. They are awesome kids.

- Windowless hallways and sterile environments prevail in our hospital.
- You'll see kids who look very sick.
- You'll see kids who don't look sick at all.
- There are serious-looking doctors and nurses.
- There is kindness everywhere.
- You may hear protesting and crying before, during, or after shots, IVs, and labs. Or just because a child doesn't feel well.
- It can be eerily quiet.
- We may need to step out if our oncologist comes by. Feel free to keep on playing with the kids while we are gone.
- Please be prepared for a brief visit if something comes up.

What You Can Bring To Your Visit:

- A happy mood and a willingness to have fun and ignore the surroundings. Please don't say how "awful this is" or "we couldn't do it." We know and are choosing to ignore it today and to be with you!
- Yummy snacks (Give them a list)
- Fresh flowers (let them know if your hospital doesn't allow them)
- Coffee or tea
- A new toy or movie for my child to open later
- A game all of us can play
- Healthy lunch or dinner to share from home or takeout and a picnic blanket. Please check with us when bringing

food because some medicines make eating rich foods difficult.

- If our kids are playing and having fun, invite me to take a break. Thank you!

- A willingness to be flexible. We will strive to have you come during a good time, but things happen. Please know we love you and don't take it personally.

Some friends and family worry about what their child will think when they visit a hospital. Well-meaning parents may be concerned that seeing sick kids will scar their child for life. That was never our experience. Children are wiser than we give them credit for, and seeing their friends in any state during a hospital visit is way better than imagining the worst. Cecilia's bestie, Tegan, joined her for all sorts of events at the hospital and loved every one of them. Those activities also gave me a chance to vent to Tegan's mama, Nikki, or take a walk and put my face in the sun. Nikki notes that we asked them to stay away if they exhibited cold symptoms, and wash up constantly, and most importantly, she says, we told her "to just be yourself and not to be all mopey." Tegan was simply herself with her bestie and that's the beauty of being four—they just had fun, even in a hospital setting.

💡 Toolbox Tip:

Share your activity, or a meal with friends outside or in a cozy corner beyond the hospital room walls. It's restorative to leave that space and be with others.

When something fun is happening at the hospital, like egg decorating during Easter time, or a visit from a clown, ask a bestie to join your child so they can continue to make memories.

Make Friends With Everybody

Although your situation certainly occupies your mind, everybody has a story and is going through something. Take the approach of treating everybody with extreme kindness when your child is admitted, especially your nurses and those helping you out in any way—bringing meals, cleaning your room—everybody. It's a great opportunity to teach or reinforce manners with your child since your room will be a revolving door with your medical team, food services, cleaning, and other people constantly moving in and out caring for your child.

> 💡 **Toolbox Tip:**
> Will there be times when either Mama Bear or Papa Bear needs to come out? For sure. Sometimes that's totally necessary. As your child's #1 advocate, you are the one ensuring that the drug dose is correct and administered at the right time, ensuring they get a solid nap, making sure their meal is correct. Most of the time that can be accomplished conflict-free. But, if you need to be a bear, growl.

Overall, I found that kindness given freely in a hospital setting comes right back to you tenfold and makes the whole adventure brighter. So, when you can, be nice.

Involve The Sibs

It's important to involve your other children in hospital parties. Having a sibling in the hospital can be terrifying, even to little ones. Since treatments are typically several months or years long, it's wise to normalize this experience. Talk about it in an age-appropriate, open way and, for God's sake, keep a positive spin. "Cecilia is getting medicine to keep her healthy" was our standard response.

Here's a "don't." Plenty of times I heard parents say, "Your brother has cancer, and he's sick. Be nice." Ouch. If you act stressed and scared, they will be stressed and scared all the time. You'll read much more about sibling relationships during cancer in Chapter 12: Your Sunshine Therapy.

Be sure your other kids get to attend their own important

activities with a trusted friend or one parent on hand. When their day is open, have them stop by for a visit to watch a movie or play a game so siblings and the family can just hang out.

💡 Toolbox Tip:

If you have older children who tend to be very busy with school and other activities, have your favorite takeout delivered to the hospital so you can create some sense of family during hospital stays at dinner time. If your hospital isn't close to home, schedule a Zoom or FaceTime at the same time every day to keep that connection going. Pick a time when you know everybody will be around, perhaps during breakfast or right before bed, if dinnertime isn't an option.

How To Bring The Party Vibe To A Hospital Stay

You've got your go-bag, great activities, and a killer schedule. Now, instead of looking at a hospital stay with dread, make plans to move in like you own the place. Obviously, be respectful of the space and any roommates, but beyond that, get creative! When hospital stays are scheduled, you can make them joyful. Here's your list for making any drab hospital room adorable.

Room Decor List:

- Streamers in your child's favorite colors
- String lights
- A lava lamp! Always a hit.
- Themed decoration kits from a party supply store, such as sports, unicorns, cars, mermaids. Cecilia's theme of choice was dinos.
- Holiday-specific fun:
  - A small tree you can decorate for Christmas and light up at night

- Diwali Rangoli sand and pre-made designs (found on Etsy and Amazon)
- Fourth of July flags
- Hanukkah wall art and make-your-own paper menorah (found on Etsy)
- Favorite framed pictures of friends and family from home
- A cute vase from home and bright-colored flowers from your yard, or have a friend bring them when they visit. (Be sure to check that flowers are allowed.)
- Classic seasonal decorations
- Music! Use an app such as Spotify or Pandora to create your own playlists. Better yet, have your Point Person assign that task to a willing friend. Music sets the mood beautifully throughout the day as much as any piece of decor. Cecilia's Songs for the Journey playlist is shared in Resources. Songs from this playlist, carefully curated to reflect our mood or to help us fire up, saved us on a regular basis.
- Small, inexpensive speaker to crank those tunes, or for calming sounds at bedtime.

You can't control everything about planned or unplanned hospitalizations. But the hospital-party mentality can go a long way toward blending "normal" life into a positive experience that might otherwise be nothing but a source of dread and fear. In doing so, you model valuable skills such as resiliency, humor, and empowerment to your child.

And who knows, maybe after a hospital stay your child will also spin around the hospital lobby, wistfully declaring, "I'm gonna miss this place!"

10

Thrive: Body and Soul
Tips for You as the Caregiver

As parents of kids with cancer, we spend most of our waking hours (and sleepless nights) thinking of, worrying about, and obsessing over every aspect of our child's body and soul. Perfectly natural. But what about you? How are you doing right now? And who's looking after your body and soul?

You are Person #1 for your child in normal times, and now you find yourself as their health advocate for a life-threatening illness. That's a mighty big undertaking. You might also be juggling a job, other children, parents, and a partner or spouse, so the idea of putting yourself first can seem selfish. Let's face it, you feel guilty taking even a moment for yourself. Right? But it's essential. Commit to putting your oxygen mask on *first* and learn to thrive, yes thrive, despite your circumstances. Back in Chapter 7, we learned how important it is to become your child's advocate. Now I'm going to teach you how to advocate for *yourself*. Let's get to it.

In the early months, my husband and I had a terrible time being there for each other when one of us was having a meltdown or felt sick. Why? We were so focused on giving everything to our kids that our tanks were totally empty, and we had nothing left to give ourselves, much less each other. We just didn't have the bandwidth to take care of another person, no matter how much we loved them. But the truth is, both you and your child need love and attention, especially as you fight something as big as cancer. When you hyperfocus on only your child's needs for three months, a year, three years, without taking time for self-care, life becomes unsustainable.

Without regular self-care, your emotional and physical health suffers, and you lack the energy to give to your partner, friends, family, or yourself with compassion and grace. All of those relationships become stretched and strained when you don't take care of yourself with that same compassion.

I learned that the hard way early on when constant stress and anxiety negatively hijacked my mood, sleep, and my ability to make sound decisions. My lack of self-care rendered it impossible to even begin to identify the good in my life because my tank was empty. All I felt was despair.

Friends and family intervened, reminding me that I had to keep up my mental and physical strength. Slowly, I found the tools for crafting moments of regular, restorative care, not only for Cecilia, but for me. Yes, for me. These practices shifted my perspective and became the turning point for our family to find our new normal and a healthier mojo. Only when your tank is full can you develop practices for your whole family and add some fun and laughter into all of your days. That's why this chapter focuses on YOU. We'll cover self-care tips for your kids in Chapter 11.

Establishing a self-care habit can feel burdensome, especially when you are in crisis. So let me help you. I'll give you options and expert suggestions for things you can do right now to take care of your body and soul. Some ideas are small and easy to do. Others require more commitment. Some are totally free; others cost money.

All provide the opportunity for reflection and restoration and open up space in your life for new ways of thinking. I'll break these down for you in the categories of Body and Soul.

Body

Taking care of your body, especially during stressful times, is a major way to build resilience, because if your body is not strong and grounded, you will eventually break. This was something I didn't pay enough attention to as a young mother whose child had cancer. I was far too busy, or so I thought. I lacked the perspective to see that the things I could do for myself would actually make life easier. It's not that I didn't have some self-care practices. I had a fairly regular exercise routine, a gratitude journal, and an occasional massage. But it was all sporadic and not nearly enough to make an impact.

When Cecilia was finally cured, I crashed hard. PTSD hit both my husband and me in the years following her cancer treatment. Thankfully, I jumped into therapy right away, and that's when my mindset started to shift. With the help of my therapist and Dr. Doni Wilson, a naturopathic doctor, I began to see how my stress responses had led me to that crash-and-burn point. I learned to recognize the warning signs, pivot, and make self-care a regular part of my life. I'm still learning—and I'll never stop.

You're under a ton of stress right now, so my goal for you is to think about realistic self-care strategies you can use both now and throughout treatment to help you avoid a full-on crash-and-burn later. But it takes intention and a real focus on yourself to make it happen.

> When we are exposed to stress, we tend to do less to care for ourselves, when really what is needed is MORE care for ourselves in order to support ourselves through the stress. If we don't take care of ourselves, we won't be able to take care of others. I use the word 'care' as an acronym to remind us of how we can support ourselves through stress—C for clean eating, A for adequate

sleep, R for recovery activities, and E for exercise. It's important to know that it's not about perfection—it's about individualizing your self-C.A.R.E. based on your body and your needs. —DONI WILSON, ND, CPM, CNS

When stressful times occur, I begin by booking some time for therapy. If the budget allows, I get a massage or acupuncture or check in with Dr. Doni. And my daily companions are morning intention setting, nightly meditation, and gratitude journaling before bed—all free.

> 💡 **Toolbox Tip:**
>
> Dr. Doni's most recent book, *Master Your Stress, Reset Your Health*, is full of simple practices for shifting from stress to flow. If you want to take it further, look for a certified naturopathic doctor in your hometown, and if you don't have one, try online! I've been with Dr. Doni for fifteen years as a remote patient.

Self-care strategies are critical for handling my busy life and profession. When my world gets crazy, they give me the resiliency to act and move towards the light in a constructive way. My goal is for you to learn these skills now, during treatment, to avoid tanking altogether. The following are my favorite tips for your body.

Massage

Your body works incredibly hard taking care of your family in good times, requiring both mental and physical stamina. And now you are managing a complex treatment regime. Give your body the gift of time on the massage table to unwind and restore. Massage is one of the best ways to relax, detoxify your stress, and release tension in your muscles. It also raises your mood by elevating neurotransmitters in your body.

If you can swing it financially, find a regular massage therapist who can get to know your body and understand the demands of what you are going through to more effectively help you relax. That's an hour of your time that truly makes a difference to both your body and soul.

💡 Toolbox Tip:
If money is tight, see if your town has a massage training institute and benefit from a relaxing treatment at a fraction of the cost by a therapist in training. In California, in 2025, 100 minutes is $25.00!

Move!

Daily exercise has a major impact on your ability to handle stress and there is no need to make it complicated. Walk, hike, roller skate, dance around the room—whatever gets you sweating and raising those endorphins. You can use exercise as your quiet time by working out alone or make it a family affair (more on that in future chapters). Everything counts, and consistency is key. If your kids are in school for part of the day, or if you have a babysitter, join your local gym and get your sweat on. Or take classes at home with apps like Peloton. Just be sure your household knows that when you are working out it's "me" time. No interruptions.

If you are the kind of person who needs motivation, there are fantastic childhood cancer fundraising organizations where you can train and raise money for the cause. Your child might even be the team honoree! While you help fund cancer research, professional coaches train you for an endurance event, like a full or half marathon, 100-mile bike ride or triathlon. With their guidance, you work on your body's individual needs and goals and get motivated by like-minded teammates.

💡 Toolbox Tip:
Our family was a big fan of Team in Training. Being a part of TnT made our journey brighter and more positive because we focused on a cause together. Arne ran a marathon (didn't love it) and biked a century (loved it), Cecilia was an honoree for the entire team, and Madi loved all the attention as the baby sister. Arne raised

$30,000.00 and got in serious shape. Inspiring. And a win-win for everybody.

Nutrition

I'm going to keep this simple for you because in the next chapter, I speak at length about nutrition for your whole family. You know the drill: Fuel your body with healthy foods and you will be in a much better position to take care of your child. Yes, your child is going through an incredible hardship on chemo and their nutrition is important. But you, as their caregiver, are also going through a lot. Give yourself plenty of healthy proteins, fats, and complex carbs, and do your best to save sugar for the occasional treat. Cut your caffeine intake off by two pm to ensure a more sound sleep.

Toolbox Tip:

- Pre-cut a salad once a week. Sundays are my day to do this, so I will always have salad on hand. I throw on some protein and I'm good to go.

- Purge your pantry, fridge, and freezer, removing the things you just can't resist and replacing them with something a little better for you. Instead of potato chips, how about popcorn? Instead of ice cream, try frozen yogurt. My choice is a daily dark chocolate square.

- Create your grocery list ahead of time. Post it on the fridge or create a shared note online and get the whole family involved in making the list. When it's time to shop or order online, your list is ready.

- Pre-plan afternoon snacks. That way, when everyone gets hungry, bring out a container of pre-cut veggies, cheese squares, creamy dip, and pretzels. Provide small plates and let your kids create their own treat. This takes the stress off of you to create something healthy every day, and your snack is ready too!

- Always have sugar-free flavored waters on hand and call them a "special treat" for both you and the kids. Eliminate soda from your household. Better yet, purchase a Soda Stream and make fizzy water from home at any time.

Exercise and nutrition are pillars for a healthy lifestyle. But there are many more ideas for taking better care of your body on Instagram, Pinterest, or check out my list below to see if anything resonates for you. Notice how many of these activities are calming, grounding, and restorative—especially important during trauma. Most are free.

Tips for taking care of your body:

- Take time alone. Start with five minutes of uninterrupted time outside, every day.

- Seek sunshine. Vitamin D actively fights depression by increasing serotonin, the hormone key to stabilizing your mood and increasing happiness. Take your lunch outside and shoot for twenty minutes of warmth. Or, if you are having trouble sleeping, aim for that sunshine before 10am to reset your circadian rhythm. If you live in a cold climate or it's winter, consider purchasing a light therapy lamp and use it daily in the mornings. And remember, cut screen time off well before bedtime.

- Take a nightly bubble bath loaded with Epsom salts for detoxifying and muscle relaxation. Use at least 2-4 cups of Epsom salt for maximum detoxification and relaxation results. Add a drop of lavender tincture as this scent is known for its calming properties. Lavender tincture is commonly found in grocery stores.

- Yoga. There are wonderful channels on Amazon Prime, YouTube (for free), or Peloton (for a subscription) for all ability levels. Yoga is an incredible escape and practice for both your body and soul.

- When life is particularly intense and the kids are asleep, look up "restorative yoga" on YouTube where you'll find professionals who will guide you through an incredibly blissful and therapeutic form of rest. There's no need for special gear. Links to my favorite teachers are in Resources.

- Take a walk. No matter what the weather, take yourself around the block or the hospital several times a day. Maybe walk every Friday to your favorite coffee shop and back and treat yourself to a healthy green tea.

- Seek out furry friends. If you have pets, nothing beats a cuddle for decompressing and lowering your blood pressure.

- Get to your labs or other appointments on foot or bicycle when possible to get your steps in. Maybe find a used bike trailer for the little ones.

- Walk on the beach or in the grass, barefoot when possible. This is known as "earthing" or grounding, and many believe it to be healthy for your whole body.

- Set a date with yourself or a friend for a weekly walk—in nature if possible. A quiet walk can be calming for your mind, and a walk with a friend can be a wonderful distraction.

- Play! Playing catch or tag in the backyard or biking to the park can be something fun and full of laughter for you and your whole family. It also gets your heart rate up.

Soul

Nurturing your soul is as important as caring for your body during a crisis. We can work out all we want or take copious classes at the gym. But if we are not also tending to what is going on in our hearts and minds, we can't reap the benefits . . . and the stress continues. For me, the three most impactful tools during our cancer years were establishing a gratitude practice, focusing on my mental health, and cultivating my faith. What's best for your soul is very personal, so I'll give you a list of additional ideas to get you thinking about what kind of soul work would lift you up the most.

Gratitude

For me, working on my soul started right at diagnosis when I happened to catch an episode of Oprah where she encouraged her audience to start a gratitude journal. I thought, *Right NOW?* What exactly do I have to be grateful for when my kid has just been diagnosed with cancer?

A gratitude journal turned out to be a life-changer, grounding me in the present and forcing me to look for moments of light and joy in my day. I still write in mine every night and the results are amazing. I exhale deeply every time I finish writing, even on my most difficult days, because it reminds me there is still good in the world when you choose to look for it.

> Consciously cultivating an attitude of gratitude builds up a sort of psychological immune system that can cushion us when we fall. There is scientific evidence that grateful people are more resilient to stress, whether minor everyday hassles or major personal upheavals. —**ROBERT EMMONS**

> Other experts in the field back this up, saying, "Noting your gratitude seems to pay off: Studies have found that giving thanks and counting blessings can help people sleep better, lower stress, and improve interpersonal relationships." —**ALEX M. WOOD, et al.**

⚲ Toolbox Tip:

Pick out a journal that makes you feel good when you pick it up. Set it up with a favorite pen by your bed. Each night, jot down five simple things that were good about that day. For example:

• A super-hot cup of tea

• A particularly good lab draw

- Laughing with your friend
- A cuddle with your child
- A day without tears

It's common to think that joy occurs only when things are going well and we have enough stuff—money, health, friends, fabulous vacations, and certainly no cancer. Only then will we truly be joyful. Sound about right?

But joy isn't always big. Through our cancer crisis, I learned that the most joyful moments, once you start to look for them, are so simple. The perfect cup of coffee. The warmth of a cat in your lap. The way the sun streams across your classroom at 9am. A hug. When you recognize small things in your gratitude journal during hard times, you strengthen your resilience, because you understand that joy is always there, no matter what. Sometimes you just have to work a little harder to find it. So do the work by setting the intention to find a little joy in your world every day.

Mental Health

Suffering is inevitable... but how we respond to that suffering is our choice. —**DALAI LAMA**

When bad things happen, it's not just the situation that makes you miserable, it's also your reaction that makes any situation worse. When we fill our minds with negative thoughts and images and let our anxiety run wild, we suffer. But if we wake up and choose to set the intention to find the good, the light, the joyful things in our day, we shore up our mental health because we counterbalance negative thoughts by filling our mind with good thoughts instead. But this takes intention and practice. For me, that work came in the form of therapy.

Our local childhood cancer support group, Jacob's Heart, had an incredible program called Art from the Heart. Volunteers helped our kids play and create beautiful art while processing their feelings, and we benefited greatly from concurrent free couple's therapy. With Marlene, our beloved therapist, we cried, vented, processed, and sought solutions to bring us together versus tearing us apart. One of the main things we learned from therapy was the concept of surrendering and acceptance, and the power of finding both in our lives.

> Acceptance, it must be pointed out, is the opposite of resignation and defeat. —**DALAI LAMA**

After the first month of Cecilia's cancer treatment, I was burned out. I couldn't see or understand how we were going to make it through two-and-a-half years of treatment, let alone another week or another day. Through therapy, we learned that accepting that she had cancer and surrendering to the reality that she would be in treatment for a long time, was the first step in finding our coping strategies. Therapy, during treatment and after, gave me a safe place to be, permission to process the grief, and a plan of action. It saved me. Through many sessions, lots of tears, and allowing myself to grieve for what we had lost, I gained strength.

That's key—you must grieve what you lost; the future you were planning, the life you were living—in order to move into acceptance and surrender.

> Some things were better in my life, such as being more intentional and mindful, feeling more secure in myself, and knowing how to take really good care of myself. And some things were worse, such as chronic low-level fear that it would come back. But by totally accepting everything, I was able to move forward. Naming that process 'grief' just like I have grieved other losses, was pivotal for me. —**BROOKE**

Even now, when difficult moments come up, I remember much more quickly that the surest way out of my suffering and anxiety is to surrender and accept life as it comes . . . life situations such as my dad's cancer diagnosis and death, a landslide into our house, COVID-19 lockdown. Only after I surrender to reality and accept my situation can I face forward, take a deep breath, and come up with a new way of living. An action plan. You can too. Try it and feel your resilience rise.

> 💡 **Toolbox Tip:**
>
> - Therapy comes in many forms. Start with your hospital's child life services team to see if there is a free local support group for you or your family.
>
> - If you are already in therapy, recommit to a regular schedule. Don't do this alone.

Remembering your Positude is another way to focus on mental health, so actively look for positive people and be mindful of the content you consume. Choose to listen to the news once a day, limit your cancer doom scrolling, and be aware of how often you engage on cancer message boards. Yes, they can be a tremendous source of help and comfort, and they are also terrifying because very real, very dark situations are shared—even children's deaths as they are happening (this really happened to me once). Take breaks and be strategic about your engagement.

You will lose friends on this journey. Usually these are people who can't handle watching you and your child suffer, so they leave. This is hurtful, but a blessing in the long run, so let them go. If friends can't be there for you in all circumstances, you don't want them in your life. Avoid those who are consistently toxic or negative, as you don't need anyone reminding you of your situation. Instead, surround yourself with bright humans, helpful people, and joyful souls. They might be your current besties, or a whole new crew. Be open to the love that unfolds and stick with those cultivating their own Positude.

Faith

If you believe in something greater than yourself—God, Buddha, Bhagavan, The Universe, or Mother Nature—you can lean into that faith when surrendering to this diagnosis and treatment, gaining the perspective, guidance, and power of whatever and whomever you believe in. If you have a faith practice, it's important to remember that your faith, your God, didn't give your child cancer. You are not being punished. Your faith is there to lift you up, to give you hope, and to fill you with strength.

> ### ⚲ Toolbox Tip:
>
> Tap into your faith daily for the biggest impact. Remember, it's a practice. Quiet your mind right before bed or do a five-minute guided meditation with your morning coffee to set a positive tone for the day. Even the smallest children can learn not to disturb their parents for those precious minutes. Mine did. And they grew up to fall in love with their own need for quiet time.

Use faith to help you surrender and accept the facts of diagnosis and treatment and stop "what if-ing." You'll find that without the constant negative mind-chatter, space opens up for more positive thoughts. Suddenly, you have the bandwidth to focus on creating your new normal, to advocate for yourself and your child, and to take better care of your body and soul.

More ideas for taking care of your soul:

- Time alone. Start with five minutes of uninterrupted time outside every day.

- Meditation

- Wake up and set the intention to find joy.

- Use an app such as BetterHelp or Talk Space to find just the right therapist.

- Draw a bath and put something lovely in it—bubbles or salts. Light some candles. As you indulge, set your intention for the next day, and say it to yourself; say it out loud.

- If you have a cancer support group for your child, remember that they often have the help caregivers need right on site to give you a break.

- Plan something fun. When friends volunteer to help, ask them for a once-a-week date night for just you, or you and your partner. Walk on the beach. Get a massage. See a funny movie. Detach, detox, and come back home stronger than ever.

Setting Boundaries

Your body and soul are telling you it's time to take care of yourself—you've got a plan and you're ready. Good job! Key to a successful shift towards regular self-care is the practice of setting boundaries because if you don't have the time, space, and support to make those changes to your life, it's unlikely they will stick and become habitual.

This can be tricky, especially for moms (or the primary caretaker), who tend to make themselves available for every single issue, big or small. This is not sustainable, especially during a traumatic life experience like cancer treatment, and it's likely you are feeling the drain of being everyone's main person right now. It's human nature to want to be there for people, but we can become addicted to this role as it boosts our ego when we feel our job is critical and nobody else can do it. But truth be told, our kids and our partners will do just fine when we take a break. In fact, by watching you put yourself and your quiet time first, you may enable them to learn to do the same.

I understand all too well the difficulties of carving out a minute with little ones running around. Heck, I can remember a time when it felt like I couldn't even go to the bathroom alone! But when I truly crashed and burned with PTSD, I had to make changes. One of the first traditions I started (and continue to this day) is my morning quiet time. After I get up, I make my tea and head to my deck (unless rain moves me to an inside corner) and I take five to ten minutes to read something that's spiritual, motivational, or inspirational.

This tiny self-care moment was a huge shift for me because I'm the family organizer and a chronic director (and one by trade!), so it's a challenge for me not to be in charge. But you know what? My sweet husband was more than capable of handling mornings solo. Even the hair braiding. We talked and set up a new system where he took on the morning routine of breakfast and getting the kids off to school, while I took on the afternoons and dinner time. Each of us got some time to ourselves that we could count on.

💡 Toolbox Tip:

If a morning meditation sounds good to you, select readings that you find inspirational and nurturing. I am a practicing Methodist, but also a firm believer that all religious leaders are actually giving us the same messages. So, I read (and re-read) a variety of faith and joy inspired material such as:

- Eckhart Tolle's *A New Earth*
- Sarah Young's *Jesus Calling*
- Thich Nhat Hanh's *Peace is Every Step*
- Dalai Lama and Desmond Tutu's *The Book of Joy: Lasting Happiness in a Changing World*

Did it take a minute for my kids (then ages twelve, ten, and six) to let Mommy be? Of course it did. I can remember quite a few times when little noses were pressed against the window watching and waiting for me to be done so they could get their mom back. My husband was critical for helping me set and keep this boundary by gently nudging them back to the breakfast table and hair braiding, handling it all with ease. My kids quickly learned to never ever interrupt this time. To this day, all of them crave and carve out their own precious alone time. Even when their dad was away, the kids knew those five to ten minutes were non-negotiable for me (unless the house was burning down). Are you parenting alone? Consider rising fifteen minutes before everybody else (and going to bed fifteen minutes earlier) to capture your calm before the storm time.

My mornings were, and are, a lifeline for starting my day centered. I don't talk to anybody and never turn on music or check my phone until my morning meditation is complete. It gives my body and mind a chance to settle into the day without starting it like being shot out of a cannon.

What boundaries do you want to set for self-care? An hour for a workout? Thirty minutes for evening yoga? Fifteen minutes for a post-dinner walk? Figure out what kind of self-care is most beneficial to you, what boundaries are needed to do it, and discuss both with your family. Then make it happen.

Taking time to figure out what you can do to help your body and soul is your ticket to coming out of this journey intact, both mentally and physically. And a centered, happy parent will increase everyone's Positude during treatment.

There is no question that these years will take their toll on you, but by actively seeking out body- and soul-filling activities—even just a few of them—you can eventually get through treatment and restore your life in the process. Will life ever be the same? No. But it can be better. These cancer years, with care and attention to your body and soul, can become merely a chapter of your life, instead of the whole novel.

11

Thrive: Body and Soul
Tips for Your Child

C hapter 10, which focuses on care for the caregiver, is required reading before you start focusing on your child in this chapter. I'll wait right here . . . Done? Great! Your oxygen mask is on first, and now you're ready to hear some strategies for helping your child's body and soul stay strong and heal during and after chemo and radiation.

Although self-care can feel selfish to adults, it never feels that way to a child. To them, self-care, like love, is nurturing. And it feels right because it is. We are designed to go hard, then recoup and recover, play, and indulge. And the youngest among us know this to be true and do it intuitively.

For children, taking care of their body and soul can simply mean giving them space to do their own thing, without interference or time restrictions. It might look like having a bubble bath for an hour, playing outside until dark, or reading a book in their cozy tent all afternoon. And they deserve it, especially when they are managing cancer treatment on top of normal life. Beyond giving them space to rest and restore, you can take care of your child's body using specific tactics to manage side effects which can potentially help the drugs do their job and leave your child's body faster.

I've curated this chapter with things you can do right now, no matter where your child is in the treatment process. Some ideas are small and easy to do. Others require more commitment. Some are totally free; others cost money. All provide the nurturing and care your child needs to survive and thrive in treatment.

Body

Your child needs help to support their body as they go through treatment and kick cancer's butt because the treatments designed to cure them also wreak havoc on nearly every other aspect of their physical health. Vincristine can cause severe bone pain; steroids can cause avascular necrosis (bone tissue loss), and all treatment protocols and cancer itself cause inflammation, possibly resulting in muscle loss. Be sure to ask your medical team for a full list of side effects for your child's protocol, then research those online.

An easy way to take care of your child's body is with an at-home massage from you. Massage is a proven stress and anxiety reducer. It can alleviate aches and pains, and it greatly improves circulation, so drugs are more quickly eliminated from the body once they have done their job. That reduces the chance that the chemo or radiation will stick around and do unnecessary damage. Massage makes a huge difference by helping the body metabolize the meds while making achy muscles feel better and reducing stress and anxiety.

> 💡 **Toolbox Tip:**
> YouTube is loaded with tutorials on massage for children, so it's easy to learn how to give a simple and effective relaxation massage. Make massage a standing appointment on your child's schedule. Cecilia's "appointment" was right before bedtime

and often involved a cozy fire with the lights dimmed. When choosing massage oil, consider a lavender scent for its relaxation properties.

You can also find a professional massage therapist and make that a regular date for you and your child! It's lovely when a person gets to know you and your specific needs.

Remember to have your child hydrate, especially after a massage, to flush toxins out of their body. See Resources for links to tutorials.

Chiropractic Care

Because treatment can cause fatigue and overall joint stiffness and muscle pain, chiropractic care can help patients (and caregivers) be more comfortable and process treatment with greater ease. Benefits include:

- Mitigating headache and neuropathy symptoms common in chemo and radiation
- Reducing muscle and joint stiffness caused by medication or long stints at the hospital
- Decreasing back and neck pain and improving flexibility

Acupuncture

Long before Cecilia was diagnosed with cancer, I had found my way to acupuncture, an ancient Chinese medicine modality, for my constant allergy issues. I was hooked after a few treatments alleviated all my symptoms and I no longer needed medication. I was working under the care of Dr. Khim Choong, MSTCM, LAc, ACN when Cecilia was diagnosed, so I was well versed in the benefits of acupuncture. There was no question that I would seek out her help and expertise when our crisis hit. Below, Dr. Choong will give us more of an understanding of how acupuncture benefits those in cancer treatment.

You probably know that acupuncture involves needles, so you might think, "Is she really suggesting more needles for my kid?"

But I can assure you, they are not like the needles in the cancer ward at all. According to Dr. Choong, most people don't even feel them being inserted during their session. Acupuncture is quite common in hospitals for helping with everything from pain management to relief from nausea and as an aid to boost the immune system.

Dr. Choong, how does acupuncture work and how can it help our kids during cancer treatment?

All systems of acupuncture utilize the stimulation of acupuncture points along the meridians, where energy flows throughout the body. In Chinese medicine, Qi is the vital energy or life force that keeps a person's spiritual, emotional, mental, and physical health in balance. Any blockage or derangement of Qi results in dysfunction, symptoms of disease. When energy (Qi) flows smoothly throughout the body, all systems of the body will be balanced and function restored. It can help relieve anxiety, pain, and improve digestion and immune function.

The human body has more than 2,000 acupuncture points and they are linked through the various meridians. Acupuncture on certain points within the meridians is believed to improve the flow of blocked or stagnant Qi. Acupuncture can unblock these meridians. This restores movement of Qi and improves health. This may all sound weird to our Western ears, but in the end, it's simply another way to think about how our body works. And the results speak for themselves.

At Dr. Choong's clinic, Cecilia would lie on the table, snuggled up next to me. Dr. Choong would talk to us about what Cecilia and I were going through, or I would email her ahead of time with the scoop if I knew Cecilia wouldn't want to talk about what she was experiencing. She would always show Cecilia the needles—which are incredibly thin—and let her know where she was going to insert them. When a person has endured as many pokes as a cancer-child has, it's likely they won't feel an acupuncture needle at all because it's so thin, small, and flexible. At least that was our experience. We would then spend the next twenty-five to forty minutes reading a book together, while the magic happened on the inside.

Dr. Choong, tell us more about those needles. Is treatment stressful, especially for kids?

Although most people think of acupuncture as the insertion of needles, it is not always how it is practiced. In Japanese-style acupuncture, non-insertion techniques can be used. For babies and children, a Japanese system called ShoniShin utilizes small metal tools to stimulate the meridians. Other metal implements called TeiShin can also be used for both children and adults. Treatments are painless and effective. This system can be used for those who are needle phobic.

Even the insertion of fine needles can be done with hardly any discomfort, if any at all. Often in the treatment of children, the needles are not used. Other modalities that are used in the practice of acupuncture include moxibustion, a warming therapy using a special herb, cupping, as well as acupressure.

Cecilia, at four years old, didn't have a ton of patience to go to Dr. Choong often, but I made sure we booked a visit:

- if her immune system (ANC) was lower than normal

- after a hospital admission

- if she had a cold

- if she was suffering from any pain or nausea

I found that if I took her to Dr. Choong before she had a dose of a drug that was known to cause severe nausea, Cecilia wouldn't be hit by nausea at all. Magic.

Acupuncture is part of an integrative approach to cancer, meaning it's not trying to cure cancer. If anybody tells you that, run. A reputable practitioner uses these mind and body practices alongside conventional treatment to help patients be better able to process chemo and radiation effects.

Thank you Dr. Choong!

> ### 💡 Toolbox Tip:
>
> Some insurance plans cover chiropractic and acupuncture care. Check yours to see if it's an affordable addition to your healing plan. If you are able to add these modalities to the family budget, I suggest you use them for yourself first and then add your child if feasible.
>
> It's also worth asking your hospital social worker what's happening at your hospital with integrative medicine. Many hospitals now offer integrative therapies for their patients with free or reduced costs for acupuncture, massage, and/or chiropractic care.

Aromatherapy

Aromatherapy is the practice of using essential oils to support mental and emotional well-being. Aromatherapy has been around for centuries and works by sending scent molecules directly to the brain's olfactory center, particularly the amygdala, which controls emotions. It's a simple but effective way to influence mood and create a calming or energizing environment.

Lavender (for calming) and peppermint (for nausea) can be particularly helpful in a hospital setting. With aromatherapy, it is important to purchase high-quality organic products, so you are not inhaling pesticides.

✷ Toolbox Tip:

You can apply a few drops of essential oils to your child's pillow, add them to massage oil, or purchase a diffuser to give the entire room a lovely scent.

Allowing your child to pick their favorite essential oils can be fun and empowering! Organic essential oils are easy to purchase at Target or a natural food market like Whole Foods, so make it a date and test out all the scents, allowing your child to pick what works for them. You can ask them to choose scents that smell like "quiet", "happy", or "naptime", or ones that remind them of someplace special. Remember, a little oil goes a long way.

Naturopathic Complementary Support

Early on, it became obvious to us that Cecilia was going to need support if her body was going to be able to handle treatment. Her immune system crashed quickly, and we were concerned about what would happen if she got a cold or a fever. We'd heard horror stories about months-long admissions for illness and having to stop chemo so a child could recover.

As we researched for some way to support her body during treatment, we interviewed far too many quacks who told us they would "cure" her cancer with their vitamin, herb, or some combination. We were not interested. There seemed to be no middle ground, and no common sense as both the oncologist and the natural practitioners tended to stay in their lane instead of working together. I was frustrated. I knew something was out there to help my child process the chemo, allow it to do its job and keep her body and immune system strong.

Somewhere along the way, in a late-night Google binge, I stumbled upon Northwest Natural Health, a naturopathic clinic that works alongside oncologists at Seattle Hospital—complementary medicine. THIS was what I had been looking for!

Dan Labriola, ND is a naturopathic physician, director of the

Northwest Natural Health Specialty Care Clinic, medical director for Integrative Medicine at the Swedish Cancer Institute, and author of *Complementary Cancer Therapies* along with many scientific papers and articles. He has been in practice for over three decades and has been voted a top doctor in both *Seattle Magazine* and *Seattle Met*.

Dr. Labriola became our medical Point Person. Since he was based in Seattle, we did our initial consultations on the phone where he took hours to get to know Cecilia's case. Much to our surprise and appreciation, he wouldn't treat her at all unless it was in collaboration with her oncology team. It took three months to convince her oncologist to take the phone call with Dr. Labriola, as he was concerned and skeptical. I appreciated that. It's important to note that complementary medicine isn't something your oncology team may be familiar with, and since it's their job to cure your child, they may automatically say no out of fear. This is understandable because it can be dangerous to play with vitamins and supplements on your own. For example, something as simple and benign sounding as B9 (folic acid) turns off the well-known treatment drug methotrexate. Working with a pro is key.

Here is my interview with Dr. Labriola.

Please explain why integrative medicine (the combination of holistic and conventional therapies) helps strengthen a child's body during treatment.

> There are so many things you can do help patients getting with cancer treatment including 1) keeping them as strong and healthy as possible while maintaining quality of life, 2) making certain that nothing, including some popular supplements, is allowed to interfere with cancer treatment and 3) taking prevention steps to prevent the patient from walking down this same path again.
>
> I have been doing this for thirty-nine years now, and I am passionate about it. Chemo, radiation, and surgery

are frequently the only deal in town that can promise a cure, although it is changing.

Why can't parents just buy a supplement at the store that they read about online?

Natural medicine plays a significant role in protecting and strengthening a child while they are going through cancer. But, if you do it incorrectly, the chemo will not work. The quandary is that you have people giving advice to unknowing families.

These people often advocate extreme measures. You'll see people like this in both medical and naturopathic communities.

Children are often given things randomly by their parents and not told by their doctors that this is dangerous because the use of these modalities has complex effects on the pharmacokinetics and other characteristics of the cancer treatment.

Could you explain that more?

Of course! Pharmacokinetics is how we study what happens to a drug (including natural medicines) from the moment you take it until it leaves your body. It has four components:

1. **Absorption:** This is how a drug gets into your bloodstream after you take it. For example, if you swallow a pill, the drug dissolves and enters your blood through your stomach or intestines.

2. **Distribution:** Once in the bloodstream, the drug travels to different parts of your body, like your brain, muscles, and other organs. This varies with the particular medicine.

3. **Metabolism:** Your body changes the drug into different forms, usually in the liver. This process

can make the drug more effective or prepare it for elimination.

4. **Excretion:** Finally, your body gets rid of the drug through urine, feces, sweat, or breath.

Understanding pharmacokinetics is essential when it comes to working with chemotherapy drugs and natural medicine because it helps determine how these substances interact in a person's body, their effectiveness, and their safety. A parent simply cannot determine all of those factors without a pharmacology degree. So, giving their child a random vitamin, mineral or botanical is well-intentioned but unwise without a naturopathic professional.

Supplement safety, including label accuracy, screening for bacteria, yeasts, molds, heavy metals, pesticides, and parasites is especially important but not common with many products. Over the years, Northwest Natural Health has developed a line of supplements especially formulated for cancer patients (see Resources for more details) called Safe and Sound®. So, there are ways to meet a child's needs safely.

The final recipe for natural medicine should be a specific and personal protocol based on a person's particular drug mix.

Yes! That is what we did with you for Cecilia, with our oncologist's blessing.

Why do many oncologists seem reluctant to automatically partner with a naturopathic practitioner or to even suggest simple holistic therapies like massage or yoga?

Oncologists are sometimes afraid of naturopathic medicine and negate it from the get-go. Why is that?

 Because of a lack of understanding and learned behavior. Older oncologists have seen patients die from some alternative and functional medicine doctors claiming to cure cancer with or without chemo. A bad history can make that relationship hard.

The information gap among doctors regarding holistic therapies is huge. They are simply too busy to look at anything other than what they do!

What is the effect of a positive attitude on tolerating treatment and eventual outcomes?

It is remarkable. I tell every patient, including the ones with terrible statistical prognoses, that patients with a positive mindset and a good support system always do better. I have thirty-nine years of experience with that and there is valid clinical data that proves it. Having the right attitude is key.

How should a parent investigate getting naturopathic help for their child?

First, ask your oncologist for a recommendation. There are many natural providers claiming to be experts who do not understand the complexity of the relationship between natural provider and oncologist despite making claims that they do. Harsh but true.

You can also see if your hospital has an integrative medicine or nutrition department that can help your child thrive, especially when side effects like nausea hit.

Whatever you do, your oncologist needs to know everything. Even the most cautious oncologists should be able to have an open, collaborative conversation with you about potential benefits and concerns about a natural modality. And keep your BS meter on when getting advice from Uncle Harry who cured his cancer with herbs.

Thank you Dr. Labriola!

> ⚲ **Toolbox Tip:**
>
> You may have noticed that many of the suggestions for children are not in the Caregiver section of this book, but that does not mean you shouldn't partake! Acupuncture, chiropractic care, and supplementation for stress, anxiety, and immunity are critical for the caregiver too. If the budget allows, go for it.

Move!

Daily exercise has a major impact on your child's ability to handle stress and to stay healthy . . . just like you! Walk, hike, roller skate, dance around the room, whatever gets your child sweating and raising those endorphins.

Balance and avascular necrosis side effects can linger for a lifetime, so look for activities that engage your child's muscles and help them practice their balance. Gymnastic classes are a fantastic way to counteract these side effects, lessening them or eradicating them altogether because they use all muscle groups and balance on the floor, bars, or beams. Swimming and water play are wonderful, too, if your child's joints and muscles ache, because there is less pressure on them underwater.

Some drugs, such as Vincristine, can have debilitating effects, such as nerve pain, a few hours after treatment. We found that going from the hospital to a park where Cecilia could bike, skate, or play helped her immensely. If she came straight home and watched TV, the pain increased significantly. Get your child to move and sweat after a treatment with something they find irresistible and fun.

💡 **Toolbox Tip:**

When your child's labs show that red blood cells are low, they may tire or get cold more easily, so pick your activities wisely. Also, when the total neutrophil count is super low, have their play time be with family instead of strangers, as you are likely able to gauge your family's health more easily. Total neutrophil, or ANC, is the body's immune fighting marker. Chemo brings down your child's natural ANC, so it's wise to be familiar with this number and understand when it's too low to be out in crowds.

Nutrition

I know it's hard. Personally, there were days when I just wanted caffeine and dark chocolate intravenously 24/7. And kids can be an even bigger challenge, especially when they don't feel well and refuse to eat. Our instinct is to just stuff anything in their mouths to rack up the calories. I've heard from many parents who struggle with this, some resorting to giving their child sugary, enticing treats just to get some calories on board.

And when we are stressed, we love dessert, right? The sweet, salty, yummy stuff. Yet the truth is that (as we were told by our oncologist) "sugar feeds cancer." Cancer cells wreak havoc by doing one thing extremely well—replicating like crazy with their super-fast metabolism. Sugars are high-octane, low-cost fuel for cancer cells to feed their extreme metabolism. Yikes.

I don't know about you, but that concept scared the shit out of me, especially since all we wanted to do was give Cecilia something to make her feel better—a treat, an ice cream, a donut . . . I felt responsible and overwhelmed. Then I realized, "Hang on, this is something I CAN control," and that felt good. The slow realization that food could be fuel for the fight, strengthening Cecilia's body to handle the rigors of treatment, was empowering. And we quickly realized it would help us handle the stress too. Healthy fats, great protein, dark veggies, and yummy fruits would enable us to thrive and stay strong. We wouldn't allow sugar to interfere with her health. You'll want to do the same, and remember to have your child hydrate, hydrate, hydrate.

You are at war with cancer, so think about what you put into your body, and your child's, as fuel for a battle. Eating healthfully can truly make a difference in your mood, keep your immune system strong, and change the negative effects of stress on your body.

Now let's get to simple, tried and true Toolbox Tips for nutrition.

♀ Toolbox Tip:

- Purge your pantry by removing the things your child just can't resist and replace them with something healthier for everyone.

- Pre-plan afternoon snack time on Sundays, and when everyone gets hungry, bring out a container full of veggies, cheese, creamy dip, and pretzels. Provide small plates and let your kids create their own treat.

- Always have sugar-free flavored waters on hand and call them a special treat. Eliminate soda from your household.

- Build-your-own pizza/tacos/bowls are fantastic ways to get kids excited about food, while offering them items that you know are healthy. They get to pick whatever they want, and you feel better because all the options are healthy.

With younger kids in particular, you can take charge of their diet in big ways without making them feel deprived or punished. You just have to be a little stealthy.

More ideas for taking care of your child's body:

- Give your child plenty of unstructured playtime.
- Seek sunshine. Vitamin D actively fights depression by increasing serotonin, the hormone key to stabilizing mood and increasing happiness. Head to the park often,

have lunch together outside. Remember to wear a hat. Note: Double check with your medical team, as some chemotherapy has specific indications to stay out of the sun.

- Plop your child into a nightly bubble bath loaded with Epsom salts for detoxifying and muscle relaxation. Load up the bath with toys or sit and read together with calming music playing in the background and the lights dimmed.

- Yoga. There are wonderful channels on Amazon Prime, YouTube (for free), or beginner yoga on Peloton (for a subscription) for all ability levels, yes, even young children! A family yoga practice, no matter how big or small, is an excellent way to process the day and start home time in a more relaxed mode.

- Take a walk. No matter what the weather, get outside with your kid. If it's hard to get you (or your kids) to take a stroll, incentivize them. For example, make walking the dog every afternoon part of their weekly chores, and pay them for it.

- Seek furry friends as a companion for your child. A dog or a cat can be a wonderful stress reducer.

- Take your child to the beach to walk barefoot in the sand, or in the grass. This simple act is called "earthing" or "grounding", and it is restorative for your body. See Resources for more information.

- Encourage play! Playing catch in the backyard or going to the park can be something fun and full of laughter. It de-stresses your child and allows them to just be a kid again.

💡 Toolbox Tip:

If you are looking for more in-depth nutrition coaching, check out the MaxLove Project. This incredible company focuses on educating their families about the power of food as medicine: "We're dedicated to improving the quality of life of families facing childhood cancers, pediatric rare diseases, and chronic hospitalizations with evidence-based culinary medicine, emotional health support, expert-driven health education, and therapeutic community."

MaxLove programs are in-person in California and Georgia, and are made available online for out-of-state subscribers, empowering families undergoing cancer treatment—their app is amazing. See Resources on how to reach the MaxLove Project.

Soul

The concept of strengthening a child's soul seems to hold a different meaning than it does for an adult. For us, conversations about nurturing the soul often involve a faith practice, or perhaps meditation or mindfulness. While children can also have faith and can practice meditation and mindfulness in age-appropriate ways, their soul strengthening is also driven by the ways in which we parent.

Key to keeping a child's soul light and carefree, as Buddhists suggest, is keeping *their world* light and carefree, which is challenging in a medical setting. But it can be done. I'm suggesting going beyond a faith practice or mindfulness. Strengthen your child's soul by strengthening their innate joy. Their Positude.

First, identify what brings your child the most joy. Where are they happiest? Don't look for happiness because of external joy, such as watching a movie or playing a computer game. Screen time is perfectly fine in moderation, but it mostly satisfies boredom and provides distraction (which can admittedly be helpful sometimes). But that's not a soul-filling joy. Soul-filling joy is your child doing that thing that makes them feel calm yet energized and causes them to feel genuinely safe and happy. What might that look like? Perhaps it's fingerpainting, or dancing in the rain. Maybe it's spending all afternoon sorting rocks or climbing a tree or reading away the afternoon uninterrupted.

Discover what that is for your baby.

♥ Toolbox Tip:

Struggling to figure out your child's soulful joy? Here are some ideas to get you going:

- Walk barefoot on the beach or in a park
- Make snow angels and decorate them!
- Create a huge mess baking or making art projects
- Watch bubbles pop
- Buy a new Lego set and let them build all afternoon

Marriage and Family Therapist Brandi Griffith notes: "Embracing the messiness in fun can help families process the messiness of a cancer diagnosis." She encourages us to be silly, messy, and lighthearted even as we are going through this traumatic time. "There are magical things that come from tapping into a child's soul and innate joy. Because their joy is where the soul lies." If your child is struggling with their mood, consider adding a Roses and Thorns practice to your dinner time. In this activity, each person goes around the table and shares one Rose from their day (something awesome) and one Thorn (something challenging). This can help you tap into what is soulful and joyful for them, even on their dark days.

Celebrate The Wins

Speaking of joy, an important piece of this journey is remembering to celebrate the wins, big and small. This is so important for everyone's body and soul, especially your child's. What can you celebrate?

- The end of a phase of treatment
- The end of a particular chemo or radiation that was tough on your kid

- The last scheduled hospital stay
- Halfway through treatment
- And of course, the end of treatment

💡 **Toolbox Tip:**

Celebrate Halfway, big time! We loved celebrating wins, and I clearly remember our Happy Halfway Party. I asked all our extended family to send Cecilia a card or a small gift in honor of the day, then we went to her favorite restaurant and had ice cream afterwards. So much fun!

- Help your child mark their successes along the way, like the end of radiation or of a particular chemo, by marking the days off of a special calendar. Powerful!

- Many children mark their courageous moments by stringing together Beads of Courage. Beads of Courage provides patients with different colored beads, each representing a significant procedure, poke, or treatment phase (identified by the child). Stringing these beads together on an ever-growing necklace makes kids feel seen and celebrates their wins. See Resources for more information and to get started on your own Beads of Courage necklace.

- Don't forget to register for Make-a-Wish (MAW). MAW is an incredible organization that allows kids with life-threatening illnesses to make a wish that they make come true. Make sure to let your child really think about what would bring them joy. Cecilia wanted to swim with the dolphins, so MAW treated our entire family to an incredible week in Florida at a dolphin nature preserve. They spoiled us with a fancy dinner, great accommodations, and a backstage day with all the creatures. And yes, Cecilia's wish came true as she swam with the dolphins in a private lagoon. Reach out to MAW today so you can have something truly extraordinary for your child to look forward to.

Can it feel scary to celebrate during treatment? Yes. But do it anyway. Your child deserves to feel all the wins, and it's so good for the entire family's mental health.

During our cancer years, we opted to go hard with all these modalities: massage, yoga, chiropractic, acupuncture, and complementary medicine. And we felt some sense of control, or participation, in her cancer treatment when we did so. Was it expensive for us? Yes. Do I regret spending that money? No way. And over twenty years later, the expense just does not matter. But this was our choice. Please know that if your budget does not allow for all these options, you can choose one or choose all the free ones. Just choose.

I strongly believe that focusing on what we could do—help her body safely fight cancer, process chemotherapy, and thrive—made all the difference in her outcome. And doing that responsibly and safely was key, as was communicating with our medical team every step of the way—don't hide anything!

Does that mean that if you do all these things your child will survive? No. Nobody can guarantee that for any of us. And we don't know for sure what it was that helped Cecilia win the battle with few side effects. Could it have been the free at-home massages? Of course! Or the more expensive complementary supplements? Yep. We'll never know.

But the way I looked at it was this: If I can somehow figure out how to swing it financially and it will increase her odds, I'm going to make it happen. Do the same while being careful to manage your financial future at the same time.

12

Sunshine Therapy

Aclassic children's song by the popular artist, Raffi, has fabulous lyrics about abundant love in a family and that was our family's theme song when the kids were growing up. We would belt out the lyrics every time they came on in the car! Singing them out loud made us feel powerful and safe because we knew that's what we wanted to be forever: a connected family that truly understood what mattered—love in our family.

Cancer tried its best to rip that apart. But our persistence, intention-setting, and Positude (positive-attitude) kept us grounded and committed to each other.

We learned that simply being together and holding tight was a form of therapy. We called it our Sunshine Therapy.

A note to readers: This chapter specifically addresses the issues that arise in a family with multiple children and between people in a partnership or marriage. All family units are special and unique no matter what the make-up is, so please take away what works for you and leave the rest behind. There are nuggets for everyone, in all kinds of family configurations.

In our last two chapters, we talked about how to fortify yourself and your child as a means of strengthening your Positude in the midst of trauma. Becoming centered and strong as individuals comes first, which is why setting clear boundaries around what you need is so key. Only then, with a self-care plan and boundaries firmly in place, can you focus outwardly on the relationships that matter most: those with the ones you love.

Relationships of all kinds take a back seat during treatment because your focus zeroes in on the crisis at hand and saps all your energy. Siblings of a cancer patient suffer when, suddenly and without warning, everything in their world takes second place. They are filled with fear and worry because they are often left in the dark, which makes their anxiety rise, and they simply miss you and your family unit when you are at the hospital. Kids can find themselves jealous of the attention their sibling is getting and feel ashamed of those feelings. That's quite a mixed bag of emotions for a child of any age to handle.

Learning how to carve out time for *all* your children and establish healthy communication about treatment as a family is imperative right now because all of you are dealing with cancer, not just the patient in the house. The way your family responds to the demands of treatment and how you talk about your frustrations and worries (or not) impacts how you will get through this experience. You want your family to get through this stronger, not be torn apart from years of disconnection. Statistically, relationships suffer more when a child has a long-term illness because tensions and anxieties mount over time. But there are solid strategies you can use, starting right now, to avoid becoming a statistic as a family and as a couple.

Your Family

We attended the family cancer support group at Jacob's Heart every Thursday night for their Art from the Heart program. A squad of volunteers and mental health professionals met us there, working with our entire family on emotional processing. There, we unpacked myriad issues, such as:

- How to manage big feelings and express them openly
- How to share treatment tasks, like going to labs, or holding a hand during a poke—without holding a grudge
- How to look at our fear and anger without fear and anger
- Remembering that our everyday schedule, like Madi's ballet class, or Mom's yoga, was important and needed to be planned for, just like planning for treatment days

What worked for each of us was different and age appropriate. For little Madi, art therapy allowed her to freely express her emotions and release them into her creations. She processed fear with the gray markers, joy when she drew a rainbow, and anger when she raged with a fist full of every color. She always slept well on Thursday nights after an Art from the Heart session.

Cecilia also loved art therapy, using stickers to act out stuff she needed to endure. She drew elaborate pictures and descriptions of her dinosaurs munching on cancer cells, destroying every one of them. Post-treatment, Cecilia developed issues around regulating her anger and saw Marlene, alone, for talk therapy to process what she had gone through and what she then felt. Marlene gave her an anger management box for home, and when Cecilia felt her anger start to boil, she'd take a deep breath and head to her room for "a moment." In private, she wrote down all her feelings and put them in the box. This calmed her enormously.

Toolbox Tip:

Ask your hospital social worker or a parent in the clinic if there is a family cancer support group near you and join it. Even if you think it's too woo-woo, sign up and give it a try. Participating in any kind of therapy is a win, but having a therapist who gets childhood cancer is gold.

If you don't have access to a family support group, hit the Dollar Store or a sale on Amazon and load up on the following:

- recycled poster board

- 8 x 10 recycled paper

- Crayola washable markers

- sticker variety packs

Now you have access to your own art therapy kit! Avoid telling your kids what to draw or do, just set it out on the floor, especially when they are moody, and allow them to process their emotions through unstructured artistic expression.

Siblings Only

Siblings are scared, sometimes angry, because they are not getting their fair share of attention during treatment, and they simultaneously worry deeply about what their sibling is going through. Parents can be gone for days or weeks at a time for treatments, which means that the rest of the family's schedule is disrupted or canceled altogether due to lack of help around the house. That's why it's so important to find the time to connect with your other kids, to keep them as informed as possible, and to open up conversations so their voice is heard.

When a sibling is diagnosed and treatment begins, stress and anxiety levels rise in your other children when they are forced to deal with big, scary questions:

"Will my sister die?"

"When will Mom and Dad come home?"

"Will I get this, too?"

"What about me?"

Left unchecked, anxiety can lead siblings to show elevated levels of PTSD, experience negative emotional reactions, and report being unhappy with life years after treatment ends. Just like their parents. Our baby, Madi, was fifteen months old at the time of her big sister's diagnosis, and she knew something bad was up. She would cry when

Cecilia got a "poke" and pace the house when any of us left for the hospital, pressing her little face against the window, waiting with her bestmor for us to return. Many of our friends thought we were lucky that Madi was so young and unaware—but that was not true. Kids are smart and, starting at birth, they feed off of the emotional energy in the room. Madi was no exception.

Initially, we thought we would spare Madi from the reality of our trauma, especially in the early months. Madi's initial reaction to us leaving her behind when we went to the hospital—crying jags, clinginess, overall sadness—broke my heart. Within a matter of weeks, it became clear what she was telling me: she needed a job. She taught me that children want and need to be deeply involved with everyday treatment life to normalize it. Her fear of the unknown was much worse than actually being a part of it all.

So, from then on, Madi went with us everywhere, from bike riding with her sis to labs, to holding her hand for weekly methotrexate shots in the leg, and whale breathing along with her during IV insertions at the hospital. Madi came to all the Jacob's Heart events, especially Art from the Heart, refusing to miss a Thursday night session.

I think she knew in her little body how good this was for her soul, too. It didn't matter that Madi was too young to understand all the scary details (nor did we tell her). She knew this was a family journey, and she needed to be on board. Trust your child, no matter how young, to step up. They most likely will if you let them.

Madi loved to visit her "iss" in the hospital when she was in-patient, having a great time causing general mischief or watching Teletubbies in the hospital bed during TV time. Madi felt safe seeing her sister, even in a hospital bed attached to an IV pole with chemo dripping from it, and Cecilia's mood was greatly lifted by spending time with her best buddy. They created a bond they have to this day because their relationship was cemented during this experience.

💡 Toolbox Tip:

Involve your other kids in ordinary treatment days. Being a part of a regular treatment day or blood draw normalizes the experience for everyone. And having a sibling along can be a fun distraction for all of you.

Siblings not only may want to be involved in treatment days from time to time, but they also need alone time with you, away from the constant cancer noise.

The first two months when we trekked to the hospital every day, Madi would stay home so she could get a nap, and so we could protect her from those first scary weeks living in the unknown. Arne and I took turns at the hospital or being with Madi so we could be equally up to date about treatment details. And we were each replenished with a healthy dose of Madi's toddler magic when it was our turn to stay home with her. She was our "Sunshine Therapy" and time alone with her was essential to our survival, and hers.

⚡ Toolbox Tip:

Make regular dates with your other kids so they can get your undivided attention, and you can soak up their particular love. Do not speak about cancer on these dates unless they bring it up. Let your child pick what they want to do with you.

The initial few weeks after diagnosis, you will probably be at the hospital daily (or even be inpatient) while doctors aim to get the cancer into remission. Strive to keep your other children's lives as normal as possible at home as you wrap your head around the processes and routines of your child's cancer protocol. Having a sibling around too early could be traumatizing for them because you don't know what's normal in a hospital, and you are likely highly stressed as you come to terms with diagnoses. Have them come when you are feeling strong, stable, and have a full understanding of what's going on instead of including them from the get-go when fear and tears are likely.

When it is time to describe what's going on with their sibling, take it slow, keep it age appropriate, and remember this: They don't need to see you lose it, they need you strong. That does not mean you shouldn't share your emotions—just be careful not to overwhelm them with adult worries and what-ifs.

Tag-Team Partnership

Oncologists, nurses, and medical teams excel at providing treatment for the huge number of children diagnosed with cancer each year. It's up to parents to figure out how to move through this experience in our daily lives—a seemingly impossible task during the paralyzing stress and grief of a child's cancer diagnosis.

Without direction or strategies for living in this new world, all a parent can do is focus on making it through the day. There isn't space for anything else, especially tending to a relationship. One of the objectives of this book is to help couples find their way, both in terms of treatment logistics and keeping the romantic parts alive. Let's start with logistics.

As we learned in the chapter Body and Soul, if we don't pay attention, depression, anxiety, and PTSD can creep in during cancer years. Stress naturally skyrockets and marriages can crack and shatter under the unending pressure and possibility of losing a child.

Sadly, most parents of seriously or chronically ill children don't know that their lack of attentiveness, combined with their child's illness, puts them at higher risk of divorce, even if the child's illness resolves. There's an even higher possibility of divorce if their child dies. Our medical team and therapist brought this cold possibility into focus, and it was scary. My husband and I are lovers and best friends, and we've moved in lockstep through the world since we were in high school. This statistic hit us hard. What we heard came across loud and clear: Pay attention and take care of each other if you want to make it through this as a couple.

At our support group, Jacob's Heart, we got the help we needed and developed the tools necessary to grow as a couple in trauma. During their weekly Art from the Heart nights, we saw Marlene for therapy while the girls worked on art projects with loving, enthusiastic volunteers. With Marlene, we were raw and vulnerable, feeling safe enough to really get into what scared us deeply and hash out all the issues coming up for us as a couple. She taught us we had to work hard to be co-captains on this journey while still remembering that we were also lovers and lifelong partners. It's a choice. And a commitment. Through therapy, we were able to figure out how to co-parent a kid in treatment and stay connected. That's where the concept of tag-team parenting came into play.

We met several couples at the hospital where one parent, most often the mom, did the heavy lifting. This kind of mom went to all the appointments alone and managed all the emotional issues that came up at home as their child dealt with their cancer treatment. Whenever we witnessed this situation, and eventually met the husband or partner, it was clear the relationship was suffering, as they tended to pick on one another and be generally out of sync. Being in the hospital and even doing all the weekly labs and meds is too much for one person. So, if you have the benefit of having a partner, job sharing is key. It reduces both the logistical and emotional toll that comes with doing this alone. If you are a single parent, pick a helper to take the burden off of you in ways that make your life a little easier.

> ## 💡 Toolbox Tip:
>
> Share medical and family responsibilities with your care partner. For example:
>
> - Have a brief weekly meeting where you figure out what must happen at home and at the hospital. Then enlist your support team to help you with everything else.
>
> - Tag team who is taking care of the house, of other children, and who is at the hospital. Rotate. This way, no one person feels the burden of being the keeper of the medical knowledge.
>
> - Have a shared system for administering shots or pills so no one person handles the difficult stuff. Rotate who is the cuddler and who needs to give the medicine.

- Do whatever you can to both be at major treatments or procedures.
- Get help at home.

Try your best to both be present for any medical updates from your oncologist. If possible, that shouldn't be the role of just one parent. Cancer treatment is a full-time job on top of being a full-time parent and having a full-time career outside of the home. If one person is leaned on too much, even if they are a stay-at-home parent, the whole family will crack. In therapy, we learned how to be there for each other during tough times, a practice we maintain to this day. And it is something to actively practice.

I encourage you to seek therapy options available for free or pay for them as you navigate these years, not only for your relationship, but for you. Remember, you can't be there for each other if you are not there for yourself. Not only does trauma increase relationship issues, but sadly it can create an environment for suicidal thoughts. Our nurse practitioner, Stacey, noted: "I had parents who committed suicide when their child died. Mental health is SO important, especially for the men who tend to stuff their feelings."

For more resources on mental health and the impact of long-term illness on relationships, please see Resources.

Remember The Romance Baby

Taking care of your partner romantically takes a back seat when cancer calls. It's easy to be upset and tearful, especially with those we trust the most. But being grumpy with each other won't make anything better. In the early months, Arne and I often found ourselves in random bad moods, sniping at each other for no specific reason while we held it together with everyone else.

Cancer is all-consuming, and it takes priority over everything. It's not surprising that the majority of parents see negative changes in the amount of fun they have with their partner, overall closeness, and a loss of sexy times.

Arne and I decided we didn't like that one bit. Together since we were fourteen and fifteen years old after meeting in sex-ed class (true story), we had history and years of romantic memories already in our back pocket. We knew how good we were together, and we were not ready to give that up.

We finished our first six months of treatment—Consolidation— ragged and burned out. Our parents saw this and, knowing that we were required to endure another two years of maintenance treatment, sent us away for a week, taking care of Madi and Cecilia while we were gone. At first, we refused to go. "You don't know how to get Cecilia to take her pill, get her labs, do her shot!" we declared. "We can learn," they replied wisely. And they did. That week off filled our tanks back up personally and romantically and gave us strength for the next round. This was the beginning of our shift, our coming back to each other. If your protocol has a maintenance period when life is more stable, make it a priority to take time away. Whatever you do does not need to be fancy or take a long time, it just needs to be a true escape.

In addition to striving for longer periods of rejuvenation, cultivate your partnership, day in and day out. Here's the trick: nurture yourself and your love with regular self-care moments and date nights. Yes, I know that sounds frivolous, maybe even ridiculous. But you must take care of yourself first, and then your partnership. This is the foundation for a strong family.

We had become tactical and transactional in those early months, which was to be expected. Time together put us as the priority and strengthened our ability to care for our kids. Our strengthened love then gave us the power to handle that day, and the next, and the next, together.

> ### 💡 Toolbox Tip:
> When friends and family are wondering how they can support you, ask for a regular babysitter. Your Point Person can set up a

schedule for you—all you have to do is plan the fun. Here are some ideas:

- Take a walk to a nearby park and hold hands.

- Sit at the beach together and read a trashy novel for an hour.

- Go to the movies.

- Hit your favorite pizza joint and just chat.

- If you have the energy, get all dressed up and see a concert!

This is one of the most important chapters for families to absorb and continually work on. Yes, it sucks that your child has cancer. Don't let it take anything else away from you: Set your intentions, be persistent about nurturing love in your house, give your other kids and partner time and a voice, and lift each other up with Positude daily. Do this, and your family will walk away from this experience strong and powerful, instead of destroyed and fragmented.

Cecilia got married to her true love in 2023! During our family dance at the reception, we belted out with conviction Raffi's lyrics about family love with genuine tears and joy. Our family dance included our Ellie, who was born one month after Cecilia's liberation from cancer treatment. Although Ellie was not physically there when the trauma happened (albeit in utero), that time is still a part of our collective family history. Dancing and belting out our family song, I knew without a doubt that the little family we so carefully took care of all those years ago with intention and Positude was indeed flourishing in life.

13

Looking Forward

*To choose hope is to step firmly forward into the
howling wind, baring one's chest to the elements,
knowing that, in time, the storm will pass.*

– ARCHBISHOP DESMOND TUTU

You'd think that once Cecilia's cancer was in remission, I
would be filled with relief, gratitude, and joy. Certainly,
when she was nearing the end of her two- and-a-half
years of treatment, I would be cartwheeling, walking on
water. Right?

All I felt was fear. Pesky, sometimes debilitating, looking-over-
your-shoulder fear. Because not everybody makes it.

During Cecilia's treatment, Arne and I bonded with six families.
They were our precious circle of support, laughter, and guidance.
We played together. We shared hospital rooms, sought each other's
counsel, and vented whenever we needed to reset. Together, we
laughed and cried as we sought normalcy and joy with one another.

In our precious circle, three children died. Luke, Rebecca, and Michelle didn't make it.

Kaleigh and Lauren relapsed, repeated treatment, relapsed again, and ended up with successful bone marrow transplants and a lifetime of long-term side effects.

One in six children with childhood leukemia die. It's simply the roll of a die. In our tight circle of friends, I bore witness to that cold fact when I sat by their bedsides during relapses or went to their children's funerals.

At one point, the fear was a clingy, heavy weight, so Arne and I met with our pastor to express our fears: *How can we strive for a positive future when our friends' kids are dying? Will Cecilia die too? When is the other shoe going to drop for us? Why is she doing okay, and they aren't?*

After compassionately listening to our guilt and worry about Cecilia's future, Pastor Sue said, "Have you ever considered that she's the hope?" Mind blown. I had been so caught up with worry that I had never considered this possibility.

"Maybe she's the hope" became a cornerstone for managing my mind going forward and being grateful for what was going on *right now*. She was okay. More than okay. We were in Maintenance and moving along with treatment without any major setbacks, knock wood.

Change Your Narrative, Change Your Story

If you are further along in treatment and everything is stable, it's time to adjust your thinking from me-and-my-sad-story towards a positive future without cancer. This is an active, intentional process that can have a tremendous impact on your daily life, and yes, it takes time to get good at it. In the chapter Body and Soul, we talked about the positive impact of taking time for yourself mentally and physically. Your mind is free to allow joy in, when debilitating fear and worry are intentionally pushed out. This can be a challenging emotional shift after the trauma of a cancer diagnosis and the early months of treatment because everything is so new, and the outcome uncertain. I'll show you ways to begin this process inside yourself and with some external choices in your life.

Here's the scenario I really want you to avoid if at all possible: I've spoken with parents one, five, ten, or even fifteen years post-treatment who are still living in those dark years, still wrapped in fear, anxiety and "what-ifs." They still lurk in Facebook cancer parent groups wondering . . .

"What if it comes back?"

"What if she fails math?"

"What if he's emotionally scarred for life?"

"What if she can't get a good job?"

I'm not saying these aren't valid concerns, nor am I saying I never went there with my thoughts. But honestly, I hated life when I lived in that space because it was hard and nothing constructive or actionable came from being there. If things are stable, all it takes to brighten your life is to decide to change your story and appreciate what actually *is* happening.

Yes, it really is that simple! And countless studies support this concept:

> Gratitude seems to reduce depression symptoms—people with a grateful mindset report higher satisfaction with life, strong social relationships and more self-esteem than those who don't practice gratitude. **–UCLA HEALTH**

Gratitude and a positive outlook are also shown to improve sleep, while relieving stress and anxiety. Sounds good to me. More information on these subjects can be found in Resources.

Nurture Your Inside

> When you are 'full of problems', there is no room for anything new to enter, no room for a solution. So, whenever you can, make some room, create some space, so that you can find the life underneath your life situation. **–ECKHART TOLLE**

Your life situation, as expressed above, is living with cancer. That is a fact. But it does not mean that your life situation is your *entire life*.

The "hope" conversation with our pastor made me realize I was lost in the dark side of our cancer journey and "full of problems" as Tolle notes above. I constantly focused on potential problems (she might die, relapse, or get sick), instead of seeing how good life was at this moment (she was in Maintenance and rocking it!). My self-absorption had become all-encompassing, and I had no space to give a shit about anything or anybody else. My made-up problems loomed large because I was not managing my mind. I had let it run wild with endless "what-ifs."

Learning how to let go of worries and anxieties that were not relevant anymore and instead orient myself around the present good moment was transformative. It takes both inward and outward work to make that transformation happen.

It's never too soon to start a positive mental shift if your child is doing well. And if your child is going through a rough patch, you'll need to have extra patience and compassion for yourself to identify the good things in each day. But you can do it. There is no need to wait until the end of treatment or years later to be joyful. You can change your narrative now and live in a new, positive story that is lifted by hope, instead of driven by fear.

Toolbox Tip:

- From the chapter Body and Soul: Start a gratitude journal and every morning or before bed, jot down five things that were awesome about the day. Everything counts, from getting great labs back to a piping hot cup of tea or a nice person who held the door open for you. Keep it simple. This is your homework and my most important advice—go for it and see what happens!

- When you spiral into "what-ifs", pause, take five deep breaths, and let those thoughts go. See Resources for tips on circular breathing to relieve anxiety.

- Remember boundary setting from Chapter 5? Here's a great practice: set boundaries around your exposure to negativity. For example, if the evening news stresses you out, just listen to a ten-minute news podcast each morning instead.

- Set boundaries around your exposure to negative people. You need, and deserve, to intentionally surround yourself with positive people who, in turn, lift your mood.

- Look for FUN each day. Be silly, see a friend, do Wordle, watch a favorite TikTok influencer. Find little things that bring you joy and do them every day.

- Get physical. Raise those happy hormones with a walk or workout, with or without the kids.

- When you thank somebody, really see them. Let them know how much their action or presence means to you.

- Review the Body and Soul chapter for more ideas to inspire your next step!

Try a few of these, then check in with yourself. Have I surrendered to my life situation? Your child is in treatment for cancer—that is a fact. But have you surrendered and accepted that fact? Remember, once you surrender and accept a life situation, then you have created space to take action if need be and to simply enjoy life instead of mindlessly worrying.

Your life situation is not your *life*. It's part of your life.

Focus Outside

As you work on managing your mind, remember that the key to changing your story and finding hope in the future is to be present. So, ask yourself, "Is my child okay *right now*?" If the answer is yes, breathe deep and smile! Next, focus that energy outward on something or someone else.

Shifting your focus outward is not only a nice thing to do, but it is also proven to increase empathy and compassion, and it reduces the perception of our problems. It gives us the capacity to move forward instead of getting locked in personal drama that may not even exist in this moment. Check out Resources for more data on the benefits of giving back.

Once I realized that, I was hooked and able to help newly diagnosed families get their bearings, just like Irene and Phil did for us. The desire to give back became the seed for this book.

What comes to mind for you?

Opportunities to volunteer, both inside and outside the cancer community, are abundant. One idea is to take an experience or frustration from your treatment years and do something to make this experience better for others.

During diagnosis, the attending doctor told us it would be much better for Cecilia if she did the spinal tap without going under general anesthesia. Because we didn't know our options, we agreed, which sounds ridiculous now—but you don't know what you don't know, especially on day one. The doctor and nurses were so kind and helped us teach Cecilia how to breathe through the pain, stay stock still, and afterwards she would "get to go to the TOYBOX!" This bribe was promised several times in the hours preceding the spinal tap, and my very motivated kid went for it. Not a tear was shed from this tiny three-year-old as she endured a horrific spinal tap—all for the promise of a toy box treasure.

When we arrived at the toy box and excitedly opened it up, Cecilia turned to me with wide, confused eyes. I looked in and found that this "magical" toy box was filled with hats . . . hats for kids who were going to go bald. As newly diagnosed parents, it was a gut punch. Cecilia crumpled into a puddle of tears.

I was incensed.

I vowed then and there that no child at Clinic D would ever experience that again. Not on my watch. Once I got my bearings with treatment, I knew what I could do to help. At the school where I teach, I co-direct a choir that tours in our community every December to bring joy to those in not-so-joyful situations. So, for the next twenty-six years, my students brought their holiday songs along with two gifts for the Clinic D toy box. Long after cancer was a driving force in our lives, this connection gave our entire family purpose as we knew from experience how important those treasures were to the kids.

Where can you make a difference?

💡 **Toolbox Tip:**

- Regularly fill up the treatment toy box. If you annually host a party, instead of guests bringing food or a gift, ask them to bring a toy for the hospital toy box!

- Create your own welcome email or text. When you see a newly diagnosed family, reach out and give them a lifeline.

- Establish a trust fund to give post-treatment kids a year of a new hobby. A family at our hospital did that, and Cecilia found a lifelong passion for horses through free riding lessons for a year after she completed treatment.

- Have flowers or cookies delivered to the nurse's station on the anniversary of the end of your child's treatment.

- Consider having your child be an honoree for Team in Training through the Leukemia and Lymphoma Society. This awesome organization raises money that goes back to cancer research. Being an honoree for a run, walk, marathon, or century riding team is super fun, and the people involved take great care of you and your family.

- Consider volunteering for the American Cancer Society's Relay for Life. Relay for Life is a volunteer-led experience uniting communities to celebrate cancer survivors, AND remember loved ones lost to cancer. ACS raises funds to improve the lives of people with cancer and their families through advocacy, research, and patient support.

Relay for Life became a family affair for us. Cecilia, Arne, and I all rotated being our local relay's opening inspirational speaker.

Arne volunteered at every relay and eventually ran our local

Relay for Life. I gave back by singing with a band to entertain the participants. Use your gifts and talents to give back! See Resources for more info on both organizations.

- Have several copies of *The Cancer Parent's Handbook* on hand. When you see a newly diagnosed family at the hospital, give them one accompanied by a hug.

- Do you have a super friendly dog? Consider going through pet therapy training for hospitals and bring your pup to children and adults in need of a soft cuddle.

Making Lemonade

I met so many incredible people during our cancer journey who have gone above and beyond in the giving-back area. They took the bitter lemons in their lives, made beautiful lemonade, and shared it with the world. Here are just two for inspiration:

Omar's Dream

While writing this book, I had the privilege of meeting Jamila Hassan, founder and president of the Omar's Dream Foundation. She lost her son, Omar, to childhood leukemia after a brave fight.

When he was in treatment, spending long days and weeks in isolation, he craved connection and particularly wanted to go back to school. Omar's idea was to set up a system where he could go to class daily, connect with his friends, learn, and forget about being a patient for a little while.

Today, Jamila has taken Omar's Dream and created an incredible foundation that enables hospitalized and medically supervised children to attend school remotely, allowing them to stay connected to their teachers and classmates. Omar's Dream Foundation funds Omar's Dream Program, which is free to qualified students and their educators around the country.

Omar's legacy is strong—thanks to his mom—as his dream of connecting kids in treatment to their communities is alive and thriving.

The Deep C Podcast

I had the joy of working with Sam Taylor, creator of The Deep C Podcast, as a guest on her show in 2024. Sam is a fierce warrior mama, whose own child endured cancer.

During treatment, Sam, like so many of us, felt afraid, isolated, and mad as hell. She did something about it by creating The Deep C Podcast. On her show, families, caregivers, friends, and community members who are supporting a child through a cancer diagnosis will feel the love and support of an open conversation. Sam notes, "Our conversations will match the ones you're already having in your head. No topic is off limits, no fear kept hidden. We speak to parents and caregivers at every stage of a diagnosis—families whose child has no evidence of disease (NED) and families who are bereaved—diving deep into their reflections and personal accounts of how they walked (sometimes crawled) through their child's cancer diagnosis."

What a gift!

Consider your gifts and talents and get out there and help others. Go make a difference! And if giving back within the cancer community is stressful for you, pick another way to give back, one that plays to your strengths. Do you love to read? Volunteer at your local library for story time. Do you enjoy being around the elderly? Volunteer at a retirement community.

Work on managing your mind with the toolbox tactics above and change your negative narrative into a positive one by helping others. Give it a try, and watch your new life story, one without cancer as the leading character, unfold.

And when the inevitable fear and anxiety creep in, you'll know how to push them aside and hear what our pastor told us: *Maybe she's the hope.*

14

Survivorship Begins Now

I am not what has happened to me.
I am what I choose to become.
CARL JUNG

I f you are reading this book, it's likely that you are early in the treatment process and not thinking at all about the concept of aftercare and survivorship. Being a survivor means it's over— you won, right? Because you are reading this book right now, you are likely facing many more months or years of treatment. I know being a survivor can feel like a dream.

At the beginning of our journey, I remember being reluctant to even say the word "survivor", and after we lost three of our little buddies to the same or similar cancer, I didn't feel like I had the right.

Survive.

That's what we all want, right? For our kid to survive this terrible thing, this cancer that has come into our lives. But I ask you—*is* that all you really want? For them to survive? Pause and think for a minute and I bet you'll say something to the effect of "Hell no. I want them to THRIVE too!" Cancer takes so much away from our children with its harsh realities and daily invasions in the form of endless pokes and prods. The reality is, current treatments leave patients with a host of long-lasting neurological and physical side effects, some very serious and scary. Here's the key and, sadly, a missing link in most of our hospital systems: Parents need to understand these side effects before they create lasting damage; you want to, in collaboration with your medical team, do whatever possible to lower their impact, and hopefully—as was the case for us—remove most of them altogether.

That is the focus of this chapter: to teach and encourage you to change your thinking about survivorship and help you become aware of the tools you have available to you now, regardless of your hospital's survivorship programs or lack thereof.

We want the best possible long-term outcome for our children—above and beyond killing cancer. That means you need to change your idea of when survivorship begins.

Survivorship begins on day one.

Currently, most hospitals do not have a practice for discussing long-term side effects and the things we can do as parents to mitigate them early in treatment. Nor does the U.S. have any kind of system-wide education for long-term side effects and appropriate interceptions as our children age. If you Google "long-term side effects for ALL", you will certainly get a long and comprehensive list because the medical community recognizes common issues that arise with certain drugs. What's missing is what to do about it. Too often, parents don't even learn about potential side effects until it's too late. Or they hear about the possibilities early but stuff the information deep inside and focus on maintaining remission. Neither response is effective.

Let's say you have a three-year-old with ALL who's taking methotrexate. This well-known drug changed the course of ALL outcomes when it was discovered that administering it in cerebral spinal fluid drastically changed the outcome for the better. The survival rate for ALL in the 1960s was less than ten percent and today, it is over eighty percent in most cases. However, that comes with a cost. Methotrexate kills brain white matter. Period. And that's serious.

White matter plays a huge role in helping the body process information. It connects the regions that send and receive signals. It affects a child's ability to problem-solve, focus, learn, and stay balanced when walking. We can't change the fact that some chemo, such as methotrexate, will impact your child's brain. However, if your child is under the age of six, their brains are still malleable and can be rewired. And while you can't undo the damage, you can change their wiring by increasing activities that facilitate balance and walking.

Remember when our oncologist told us, "She'll never do math or science" because of the side effects (often called late effects)? If we had simply listened and stuffed that comment away, Cecilia may have had a host of neurological issues common to those with childhood leukemia, because he was right! Chemotherapy treatments can greatly reduce or eliminate a child's ability to do math or science. Why? Because late effects can include slower processing speeds or may impact executive functioning, planning, attention, as well as the ability to multi-task. My tactic was not to give up, but to dig in. I found and called the head researcher for Cecilia's protocol and asked him all my questions. Like I said earlier, pretty bold, right? And the right move back then. While you could certainly try finding and calling your protocols' head researcher, times may have changed at your hospital. So, start with your hospital social worker and see what connections they have for ameliorating long-term side effects. Many hospitals are now well-connected with learning specialists, but you must continue to advocate for that help early and without prompting.

No one will suggest that you make that happen—remember, your doctors are busy saving your child's life.

> ### 💡 Toolbox Tip:
>
> The head researcher of Cecilia's protocol was very clear: You can't fix white matter that's been damaged by chemo. But you certainly can rewire her brain. His recommendations for her age and protocol included:
>
> - Reading constantly to your child and teaching them to read if they don't already. The earlier a child can read the less likely chemo will destroy that ability.
>
> - Focus on having them memorize math facts early.
>
> - Keep reading and math rewiring fun! We always had a reward system, and several "educational" computer games were considered a rare treat to Cecilia. She loved playing the games in Reader Rabbit and never realized she was rewiring her beautiful brain.
>
> - Be patient and work with teachers openly and honestly. (See below for school tips.)
>
> - Begin an activity that works on balance and coordination, one that is fun for your child. Be sure this does not feel like a chore. Don't tell them they have to do it to "fix their brain"—that's not something you should burden them with at any point in their journey. We gave Cecilia options, and she chose a gymnastics class and had a ball! We made it a family affair and let Madi take toddler class at the same time.
>
> - After treatment, continue these practices. Sometimes, organizations can help you with expenses, so ask your social worker. Near the end of Cecilia's treatment, we received a call from an organization that offered a free year of an activity of choice for a survivor. A local parent who'd lost a child decided this was their way of giving back and helping other kids acclimate into the real world again. Cecilia chose horseback riding. Not only did this become a lifelong passion, but that

activity eliminated potential side effects with her balance, walking, and necrosis (bone loss). Amazing. And free for an entire year!

The Conversation Is Changing

The good news is the conversation is changing when it comes to survivorship. Earlier action to address long-term side effects, and a focus on post-care treatment is a growing trend. There is so much you can do to help the chemo and radiation do their work, save your child, and get out of their body quickly.

There are some incredible doctors at the forefront of this moment, paving the way for better collaboration and information-sharing between patients and doctors. And there is energy around potentially creating some kind of standardization for information-sharing so parents don't have to work so hard to understand what kind of help their child needs.

While most major hospitals now have survivor (or aftercare) clinics, it's rarely, if ever, a requirement for a patient to join them. And families are not commonly introduced to the survivorship clinician until treatment is over.

If there is one thing I want you to hear loud and clear in this chapter it's this: *Survivorship begins now.*

Regardless of your clinic's setup, take it upon yourself to become informed by beginning the conversation with your nurse practitioner, doctor, your hospital's survivorship clinic (if they have one), and social worker. The rest of this chapter is devoted to helping you navigate this system and thrive as you advocate for your child's future.

In 2021, I began working with Dr. Stephanie Smith, a pediatric oncologist and researcher at Stanford Children's Hospital. At the time, she was interviewing survivors and their parents about their aftercare at their hospital and life experiences in the years after finishing cancer treatment. Dr. Smith's academic interests include cancer survivorship, community engagement, health equity, and patient-family-clinician communication. The goal of her research is to improve childhood cancer survivors' long-term health and engagement in recommended survivorship care.

Dr. Smith is passionate about the intersection between clinical care and clinical research and is committed to understanding the effects of childhood cancer therapies throughout a patient's lifetime. She aims to develop community-based partnerships to share evidence-based survivorship research to real-world clinical practice settings in communities. She addresses those with socioeconomic disadvantages and structural barriers to long-term follow-up care by targeting social determinants of health to improve access to care and health equity for adolescent/young adult (AYA) cancer survivors.

Dr. Smith and I have collaborated in writing for Stanford Children's Hospital as they develop informational materials for families post-treatment, and we spoke together on the Health After Cancer podcast, episode 6. Check it out!

A Conversation With Dr. Stephanie Smith

When should parents begin to focus on restoring health, and how does that relate to treatment?

I have always thought that medicine should focus not only on diagnosing and treating illness but also on restoring health and well-being. Good health is not just the absence of disease. It requires consideration from the whole family, in addition to the child undergoing cancer treatment. Kids receiving cancer treatment are still kids, and they want to play, learn, and stay active. A huge part of our role as their oncologists is to manage (and ideally prevent) symptoms so they can feel like themselves and keep doing all those important "kid" things. As parents, something you can do now is to be sure that your child's oncology team knows what your child loves to do and what activities are important for your family's overall well-being. That way they can work with you to align shared goals.

Some parents and kids wonder, "If I've finished cancer treatment, why do I need to continue in an aftercare clinic?" One of the biggest questions is, "What's in it for my kid?"

Across the U.S., there is a lot of variability in how childhood cancer survivorship care is delivered.

The recognition of the need for survivorship care has grown dramatically in the past twenty years. International recommendations are that every child treated for cancer stay connected with survivorship care throughout adulthood because some cancer treatments can have health effects ("late effects") years, even decades, after they were given.

Survivorship clinics, also called "long-term follow-up" or "after-care" clinics, are a way that survivors can access this care. Yet less than twenty percent of childhood cancer survivors continue to receive this specialized care in adulthood.

The focus of survivorship care is on optimizing health through considering and addressing the impact of cancer on physical and mental health, social relationships, growth and development, learning, school, and work. There is a big emphasis on understanding potential health risks and the prevention and early detection of health effects from treatment. This could involve screening (tests to look for issues before any symptoms), encouraging healthy lifestyle behaviors such as physical activity and nutrition, or counseling or mental healthcare to help children and families emotionally process their cancer experience.

Many families may not hear about survivorship care until after their child finishes treatment. Work is ongoing to figure out the right time to introduce these concepts and plant the idea that planning for long-term care is foundational for ongoing health.

I'd like to know about some of (this) during treatment, so we know what to expect down the road. —**HEATHER, CURRENT CANCER PARENT**

What should a family do when no survivorship program is available or if long-term side effects and aftercare is not part of the conversation in their oncologist's office?

Despite the recommendation for universal survivorship care, we know many survivors and families may not be aware of or do not have access to these specialized programs. As a parent, you should feel comfortable asking your child's oncology team where they can get survivorship care after finishing treatment.

There was no survivorship program. You just went back to your pediatrician and came back to the oncologist for blood work. No one really told us what to expect with a rebounding immune system, dealing with return to school, life, etc., dealing with trauma... The supports and services that were there during treatment were suddenly gone and you were just supposed to be ok. —**ANONYMOUS MOM OF A CHILD WITH CANCER**

A nonprofit organization, the National Children's Cancer Society, maintains a list of programs by state, and the Children's Oncology Group has another list that is searchable by city and state. More details are available in Resources.

I know you've interviewed many patients and parents about their post-treatment experiences. What's the biggest problem you're seeing?

I think one of the biggest issues is that—understandably—many kids, teens, and parents do not want to have to think about anything that has to do with cancer after they've finished treatment.

As oncologists, we too wish our treatments were less toxic. The possibility of facing potential health risks years after cancer treatment can be overwhelming and may drive people away. And there is so much variability in the type of cancer survivorship resources available to families that it's no wonder the vast majority of childhood cancer survivors stop coming back to survivorship clinics when they become adults.

From your perspective as both researcher and oncologist, what are the gaps in treatment, particularly when it comes to long-term side effects?

As oncologists, we talk about potential health risks related to cancer treatments as part of "treatment consent" discussions. Yet these discussions take place during a time of intense emotion and trauma, often just hours or days after a child's cancer diagnosis. This is not a time when much, if any, information can be retained. The ideal time to talk more in-depth about potential long-term side effects of treatment is not well known and may be different for different families, based on the treatment protocol.

Another issue we face is that childhood cancer treatment protocols are changing rapidly, always with the goal of improving effectiveness and cure rates and decreasing or minimizing long-term side effects. However, this means that survivorship research (understanding the long-term health effects of new cancer treatment protocols) lags behind because most of these effects take a long time to develop.

So the information we know today about certain medications may change in another five, ten, twenty, or thirty years, and with that, recommendations for screening and follow-up care may change as well. If cancer survivors are not still connected with their treating hospital or a survivorship program, how will they know about these new findings and changes in recommendations? This is a challenge we discuss all the time at cancer survivorship research meetings, and we are committed to trying to improve this with new approaches.

What is the one message you have for parents of kids with cancer as they learn to navigate a system currently without much structure?

Just being aware of the fact that cancer treatments can have long-term health impacts, and that research is ongoing and new findings may change today's recommendations. It's important to stay connected with aftercare programs in some way as kids become teenagers and adults. And it's important to never be afraid to speak up to your cancer care team if you're not sure whether something you're experiencing could be related to past cancer treatment.

How does survivorship change from the patient's point of view? What do parents do when their child says "no" to an aftercare clinic visit?

For many kids, their perspective on survivorship or aftercare may change over time. Your child may say "no!" or go through phases of their life when they won't want to deal with cancer at all.

Sometimes, years later, they will want to talk about it to understand more about their treatment and what it means for their present or future health.

You can be a great resource if they have questions or want information years later because you may remember parts of their treatment better than they do, especially if they were quite young when they were treated.

Thank you Dr. Smith!

A Note About Returning To School

Going back to school and aftercare go hand in hand. It can be both a joyful and a scary thing for your child to be in school during treatment or for them to return to school after an extended absence due to treatment. You might wonder, "How will my child stay healthy? What accommodations can be made for any learning differences showing up? Where can I find out how to advocate for my child's legal rights for accommodations?"

This is a complicated and complex topic. Thankfully, there are a ton of resources out there to help parents through the process (see Resources for a start). Start by connecting with your hospital social worker for advice and your school principal to see if they have ever developed an IEP (individualized educational plan) for another child. If so, they will be ready to help you from the get-go. An IEP is required of all public schools as a way of bringing together all the teachers, administration, and counselors who come in contact with your child. This is so they can develop a plan that addresses your child's specific needs both during and after cancer treatment. Students qualifying for an IEP must show evidence of a disability that affects their ability to learn. During treatment that could mean things such as getting tired easily or being unable to run in PE. Post treatment, you may find that your child qualifies for extended time for tests and quizzes. If your school has never done an IEP before, not to fear. They are required to do so and will take the time to make it happen. If your child is in private school, they tend to use a similar format.

> 💡 **Toolbox Tip:**
>
> I worked at a private school at the time of Cecilia's diagnosis, so my situation is a bit different since I knew a lot of the teachers. During her time at this school, which was K-12, her teachers, in general, were incredibly helpful. For example, the way her brain rewired itself for math meant that she could always get to the solution, but it often had to be in her own way—not the "prescribed" formula that teachers taught. Once they understood her needs and abilities, we were able to let her flourish in math in her own unique way. By her senior year in high school, she nailed AP Calculus.
>
> When we first returned to the classroom in kindergarten, Cecilia was still on prednisone. I remember telling her teacher about Cecilia and what it would be like, potentially, when she was on day five of that drug. Her eyes got big as she listened, took the information in, and then said, "I've got it." She was amazing, even when Cecilia had a meltdown from a prednisone rage. They developed the best bond. She and Cecilia are still tight today!
>
> If your child is unable to go to school in person, remember to check out Omar's Dream. This organization is changing the way that kids who are in-patient can continue to go to school with their class.

Moving The Needle

Part of my passion for this chapter stems from frustration. At the end of our treatment in the early 2000s, there were few, if any, survivorship clinics. My advocacy for addressing long-term effects was ongoing during treatment and related specifically to neurological rewiring and physical health for our child. On the last day of treatment, we were asked if we'd like to be part of a study for kids with cancer, one where we would come in once a month for labs. My reaction was simply: "What's in it for me?" and Cecilia's reaction was, "No more needle sticks!"

After two-and-a-half years of treatment and over 2,000 blood draws, spinal taps, and methotrexate shots, coming back to deliver more blood for research held no attraction for any of us. There was no upside. My, how things have changed! Our hospital now has an amazing clinic for mental and physical help that our very own oncologist, Dr. Gary Dahl, helped create. The Stanford Adolescent and Young Adult Clinic helps children thrive post-treatment and beyond—in all aspects of their lives. You'll find all the details about this awesome program in the foreword for this book. However, this clinic was not an option back then, so we passed on the monthly trips to the lab for research.

Although Cecilia fared quite well with latent effects, it was certainly not all roses for us. For example, throughout treatment, we asked if we should harvest Cecilia's eggs and were told no, the current data didn't suggest that the chemo would harm them. That decision would come back to haunt us nineteen years later when Cecilia was working for a company that was researching an at-home fertility test. She asked me again if there was any reason for her to worry about her own fertility and I replied again, "Nope! They told us there was no issue." Cecilia took the test, and we were all surprised to find out that my twenty-four-year-old had the eggs of a forty-year-old. I was furious. She was concerned. Even though love, marriage, and kids were way in her future, she suddenly didn't feel as though she had time to spare.

I quickly emailed our oncologist, who connected Cecilia with the Teen and Young Adult Clinic. Within days, she was on the phone with a nurse who was explaining the results and was able to refer Cecilia to an affiliated fertility clinic. A few months later, twelve healthy eggs were extracted and frozen. And because of her status as a survivor, she received a fifty-percent discount on her fertility treatments.

Happy ending! But was all that drama necessary? I don't think so.

> 💡 **Toolbox Tip:**
> Check out the Livestrong website which lists the fertility clinics with discounts for survivors.

My wish is for a systematized way for patients to access their healthcare information so they can receive ongoing current data regarding their protocol. Cecilia's protocol, POG 9201, was new at the time, and the little girls in the study needed to grow and mature for the data on fertility to show up. But it would have been nice to have had that information right when it became available and not have to find out by accident. And what about the other women who didn't take an at-home test and decided they would wait to start having children later in life?

Thanks to doctors and researchers, change is coming.

Standardizing childhood cancer's late effects, options for mitigating those effects, and tracking long-term testing that's needed for a healthy life is where we are headed. I can't wait.

Cecilia found a survivorship clinic near her apartment where she can receive her primary care and other health services under one roof with providers who understand her history. As a young woman, she is no longer afraid of a clinic that only promises another needle stick. She is empowered because she finally has a comprehensive collaborator in her good health, one who can track her needs, offers preventative testing, and is a teammate in her long and healthy life. One of the best benefits of Cecilia's survivorship clinic is their "passport for care"—a credit-card-sized easy reference document that lists on the front all the medications she took. On the back are specific recommendations for preventative care and screenings based on her specific protocol. This card allows her to walk into any doctor's office and immediately communicate her needs and medical history with ease. Pretty cool!

15

Love, Loss, & Living With Grief
When Your Child Doesn't Make It

Earlier in *The Cancer Parent's Handbook*, I spoke about my first friend in the cancer world, Irene, who I met in Clinic D shortly after we were diagnosed.

During Induction, in addition to taking chemo at home, children with ALL have many trips to the day hospital where they receive infusions, or heavier injections of medications, and spinal taps filled with chemo. It is an incredibly raw and awful time, as protocol calls for pounding kids with enough chemo to put their bodies in remission, hopefully for the next few years. Hopefully forever. Induction lasts at least a month. Confusion is at an all-time high in this phase for both parents and kids, as is exhaustion and worry as you try to help your child be okay with all that is happening to them.

It was during Induction that I met Irene. As I entered Clinic D for the appointment at the day hospital, eyes bleary and vacant, Irene marched up to me with one kid in a stroller and a baby strapped to her in a front pack and said, "I'm Irene. You look like you need help." I consider myself lucky that I was on deck that day, with Arne at home with Madi, because that was the day I met the most remarkable woman, who also became my friend.

Irene sat me down and began one of many pep talks about the childhood cancer world, what to expect, and what was going to happen this month. Most importantly, she shared what my options were (I had options? I did!). Her son, Luke, who was the same age as Cecilia, got restless in his stroller. In short order, the kids were bounding through the ward, causing mischief, and having fun. We exchanged email addresses and phone numbers and immediately became fast friends. It was Irene who opened my eyes to not only the need, but the necessity of advocating for our kids and for ourselves. Because Luke was many months ahead of us in treatment, Irene had it all going on and dialed in. She sent me copious notes and advice about what to expect with a certain drug, or the next phase of treatment we faced, and tips for managing both. I was hooked by her eye-opening advice and positive energy. I took her suggestions to heart, found my own kernels of wisdom along the way, and shared everything with every new family I saw walk bleary-eyed and vacant into Clinic D . . . just like Irene did for me. She was one of the reasons I wrote *The Cancer Parent's Handbook*.

Arne and I became fast friends with Irene and her husband, Phil. Phil is a rock star kinda dad and influenced how Arne approached treatment. It was more than being trauma friends, thrown together in the mosh pit. We just clicked. And click to this day.

During our treatment years together, we celebrated milestones, held each other's hands, and most importantly, were together for the incredibly dark times that came to Luke, Phil, and Irene. Luke had the same diagnosis as Cecilia, but due to unusual circumstances, his ALL morphed into something more—AML. He didn't make it.

Being with Irene and Phil throughout their journey was a privilege, as was being by Luke's bedside to say goodbye the day his body left this earth. I asked Irene if she would be the cornerstone of a chapter on love, loss, and bereavement.

Luke's journey, and how Irene and Phil advocated for what was best for him and the entire family, is nothing short of unique, inspiring, and amazing. Here is my interview with my friend and warrior-mama, Irene.

Tell us about Luke.

> Luke was named after the beloved physician who wrote the Gospel of Luke and the Acts of the Apostles. We love that Luke's name means "light giving." We were blessed that Luke was an easy-going child. He was very sociable and enjoyed letting people hold him and did not have separation anxiety. Smiling and laughing is what Luke did best. We took Luke to Gymboree classes, and he was a total fan of the parachute and singing. A Gymboree play group was formed, and it was fun for Luke to play with buddies. Luke also loved dinosaurs and Thomas the Train. He especially loved showing everyone his loud, roaring dinosaurs and brought them everywhere. He was also a big fan of watching Barney, which was a big hit at that time. Luke really loved our dogs, BooBoo and Tinker. Of course, they would let him pet them, but the minute he started pulling on their fur, they made a quick exit. Luke was a sweet and wonderful child who was always smiling and laughing.

One of my favorite memories is how Luke and Cecilia both loved and gravitated toward dinosaurs. I think they empowered the kids and made them fierce! These two were full of joy and mischief.

How did you first learn that Luke had cancer?

His brother, Jeremy, was born on July 3, 1997, and the boys were twenty-two months apart. When Jeremy was seven weeks old, he was congested and coughing, so we took Jeremy to see his pediatrician and Luke came with us. The pediatrician said Jeremy would be fine, but she wanted to examine Luke. The pediatrician looked at Luke's arms and his back and noticed petechiae (burst blood vessels) on his arms and a couple of small bruises on his back. She told us to have Luke take a blood test and that the clinic would call us back. They called and told us that Luke had leukemia and told us to bring him to Lucile Packard Children's Hospital as soon as possible.

Tell us how you and your husband, Phil, first reacted to the diagnosis?

We were completely stunned by Luke's diagnosis. We prayed and asked God to please help him heal and help us survive it, too. Thankfully, we were blessed with our family, church, and friends constantly praying for Luke's healing. But it was like our lives just exploded into chaos and massive stress that only got worse. My mom was an angel and stayed with us so we could be with Luke at the hospital.

Luke's oncologist told us they had to do a bone marrow aspirate immediately, without any kind of anesthetic. We were shocked and asked them to please numb him, but they refused. It was unbelievably heartbreaking because the bone marrow aspiration without any pain medication was brutally painful for Luke. Three nurses held him down while the oncologist did the bone marrow aspiration. Luke was screaming and I still can hear him screaming for us. After that horrible experience of Luke being traumatized, we no longer agreed to any bone marrow aspirations without some type of sedation. We regretted not demanding sedation for Luke because he deeply disliked the oncologist after that terrible experience. It was absolutely unnecessary for Luke to suffer like that.

Cecilia, too. Thank goodness sedation is standard now for procedures like that.

That was a pivotal moment for you. It was for us as well, as we had the same experience, and it was horrific. Note for readers: Advocacy begins now. Demand what you know is right for your child.

The oncologist told us that Luke had Acute Lymphocytic Leukemia, and his treatment protocol would be about three years. It was all so overwhelming and heartbreaking to realize that we were going to have to watch Luke suffer through chemotherapy treatments, but at least he had a ninety percent chance of surviving. Luke was turning two years old when he was diagnosed.

After that initial bone marrow aspiration, what changed in your parenting advocacy for Luke?

Phil and I made a promise to each other that we would read all medication labels and make sure he was given the correct blood type for any transfusions. It is so important for parents to do this and be an advocate for your child. The nurses were great, but any human can make a mistake if they are tired or rushed.

When Luke started his first chemotherapy treatment, it was really hard watching and knowing that this poisonous chemical was going through his body in order to kill the cancer cells. A normal routine with chemotherapy treatments would be that Luke would get his chemotherapy, go home, get a fever, and get admitted back into the hospital because of the risk of infection. Unfortunately, whenever he had to get antibiotics, he would get a yeast infection. When he had to start taking steroids, poor Luke had crazy roller coaster emotional outbursts and was so agitated.

Phil took Luke into the LPCH Day Clinic because Luke needed a blood transfusion. One of Luke's favorite nurses was going to be managing his blood transfusion. Luckily, Phil read the label on the blood they were about to transfuse into Luke because it was the wrong blood type. Phil and I were shocked and upset because that transfusion would have killed Luke. Even though it was Luke's favorite nurse, we called and emailed the president of the hospital and let him know what happened.

Thankfully, there was an official apology, and they wrote a letter saying there would be a more careful process, so it didn't happen again. We hope it hasn't happened again to anyone. Just remember to look at all your child's medication labels and blood transfusion labels.

What brought Luke comfort during this time?

One important thing in Luke's life was his yellow blanket. A good friend named Polly made this small yellow baby blanket for him and Luke was very attached to it. He had to have it with him at all times. One time he threw up on it and we had to wash it. He was upset and cried so much for his yellow blanket. Wonderful Polly made him a second yellow blanket, but Luke rejected it because it was not the special blanket.

I remember Luke and that yellow blanket always being attached to each other! How did you manage those early days of treatment with such a young family? Who helped you?

Luke loved being home with his little brother, Jeremy, and having family members visit. Jeremy was only seven weeks old when Luke was diagnosed. We had to be careful and limit Luke's exposure to a lot of people since he was going through cancer treatment, but we also wanted him to have fun.

Sometimes my family would take Jeremy to stay with them for two weeks so we could focus on Luke. We felt guilty having Jeremy be away from us, but we had to take care of Luke. Sometimes we would bring Jeremy to the hospital with us, and we could all spend time together as a family. We met some wonderful volunteers who would come to Luke's hospital room and ask if they could babysit Jeremy or stay in the room with Luke so we could take a break. Child Life Services had amazing employees who helped us a lot. One favorite staffer, Jeff, would walk Jeremy around the hospital, give him his bottle, and keep Jeremy occupied. Sometimes he would sit with Luke and play games and make Luke laugh. Joe was another amazing volunteer. He took care of Jeremy often and walked him around the hallways in his stroller. It warmed my heart when I would see Joe sitting on a bench and feeding Jeremy.

The front desk receptionist, Candace, was always kind to our boys and all the cancer kids, too.

I remember all those people so fondly. Truly Child Life Services, at any hospital, is a godsend for parents, siblings, and patients.

Whenever Luke had his chemotherapy, he was admitted into the oncology unit. There were private patient rooms and other rooms with two beds.

Luke started having roommates, so we met a lot of children who were battling different kinds of cancers and, of course, met their parents. Luke met so many sweet children and teenagers while admitted. It was good to meet other families and talk about our different experiences and try to help each other.

During the Consolidation phase of treatment, we started taking Luke around the oncology unit and nearby hallways in his wagon, in his stroller, or he would ride on his chemotherapy pole. He enjoyed saying hello to other cancer kids, and we met Cecilia and your family while cruising the hallways. Cecilia's grandfather, Glenn, was so sweet and he dressed up as Santa Claus for Christmas and Luke was so excited that he got to sit on Santa's lap. We made some very special memories with the Lang-Ree family.

We sure did…

You and Phil are such a strong couple. What was your strategy for taking care of Luke together?

We were blessed that Phil's employer was incredibly supportive and allowed him to take time off so he could focus on Luke, especially during the first

year of treatment. We worked things out where
we traded off spending the night when Luke was
hospitalized. We counted our blessings that Phil had
a stable job because some parents had bankruptcies
and financial problems while their children were in
treatment.

Phil has always been a great father and was
always kind and patient during Luke's journey.
Unfortunately, Phil started having severe headaches
and ended up having high blood pressure from all
the stress over Luke. We were stunned when we
found out that some LPCH parents of cancer kids
get cancer themselves and pass away during their
children's treatment. The stress is so enormous on
parents, and it opens the door for illnesses.

That's why an entire chapter of *The Cancer Parent's Handbook* **is devoted to self-care for the parents—it can't be taken lightly.**

How did you find some joy and relief during treatment?

It was such a relief when Luke got to come home
between chemotherapy treatments. My sister Diana
came to live with us for a while and she loved
spending time with the boys. We would take Luke
and Jeremy to the little local zoo and train ride as
much as possible. We let Luke ride his bike inside
some of the local malls.

One of Luke's closest friends was Alex. He had
ALL. They loved being roommates. We bought a
puppet show tent so they could both get inside and
put on puppet shows for us. There was a moment
in time when Alex's health was in trouble, but
he recovered and healed. Luke really loved Alex,

and we were grateful that he had a good buddy.
I remember taking a break while our other son,
Daniel, and Alex were napping, and Phil stayed with
Luke. I went to the Stanford Mall and sat down on
a bench and cried. It was so strange seeing all these
people happily shopping with their children while
our child was at LPCH fighting off cancer. It just
seemed so unfair.

Alex and Luke became honorees for the Leukemia
Society South Bay Running Team. The runners
would do fundraising with Alex, Luke, and other
leukemia patients as their honorees. The runners
would run half or full marathons, and some
participants walked the half or full marathons.

Parents would take the honorees to pass out water
to all the runners and cheer them on at the practice
runs. Luke loved all the attention he got from the
ladies. They all knew Luke was enjoying collecting
quarters, so some of the runners would give Luke a
quarter. It made Luke the happiest honoree.

Luke was blessed by the Make-A-Wish Foundation.
They had this incredibly fun event where they let
cancer kids fly in a plane from the San Francisco
airport to Monterey and back. There were people
dressed up as Snow White, Mickey Mouse, and
other fun characters. We were singing and all the
kids had a blast. On Mother's Day, they had cancer
families and their cancer kids for a day at Great
America. The most amazing thing that happened
was the Make-A-Wish Foundation installed a big
and beautiful play gym and swing set for Luke in
our backyard. The local news crew came to our

house and interviewed us about how excited Luke was about his new incredible play gym. We cannot thank the Make-A-Wish Foundation enough for their generous gift for Luke. Luke was able to enjoy so many fun times with his brothers on the play gym.

Managing the reactions of family and friends during cancer treatment alone, much less at the end of life, can be frustrating and exhausting! How did you handle their emotions and support, or lack thereof, while focusing on Luke's needs?

Even though most family and friends were supportive, some family and friends could not truly understand how trying to save our child from dying of cancer affected our life. We had some family and friends make insensitive comments and it was so upsetting on top of the constant stress we were dealing with. One time we spent six hours at the hospital for an appointment we thought would be two hours. We were exhausted, but we drove to Sacramento for my mom's birthday party anyway. A family member opened the door and rudely and seriously questioned why we were so late. I responded with not so nice words because I couldn't believe how this person could have no clue or compassion for us. Unfortunately, there are people in life who will be insensitive no matter what. They just don't get it. Sometimes you have to just let their insensitive comments go or tell them that their comments are hurtful. You have to realize that they have absolutely no idea what your life is like unless they are in your shoes.

How did you learn Luke was relapsing?

I was pregnant with our third child, Daniel, and he was born on May 15, 1999. Jeremy was twenty-two months old when Daniel was born, and Luke was going to be four years old. During the last month of my pregnancy with Daniel, Luke started needing red blood and platelet transfusions, which was very alarming. We were worried and stressed that Luke was relapsing. We prayed and asked our family and friends to please pray for Luke. The stress was overwhelming. We felt numb again.

Phil and I took Luke to his oncologist after we brought Daniel home from the hospital. They took a blood test and found concerning cancer cells, so Luke had to have a bone marrow aspirate the next day. Waiting for the results was unbelievably scary and stressful. The next day, Luke's oncologist told us that Luke had relapsed, but he had relapsed to Acute Myelogenous Leukemia. His oncologist told us it was rare for an ALL patient to relapse to AML. We were devastated. His oncologist told us Luke was terminal. She explained that Luke needed to get chemotherapy immediately and hopefully it would get him back into remission. She told us the chemotherapy was brutal, and Luke could have complications from it.

Phil and I made an appointment with a bone marrow transplant doctor at Fred Hutchinson Cancer Center in Seattle for a second opinion. Unfortunately, Jeremy's and Daniel's marrow matched each other, but not Luke. Since Phil is Dutch and I am of Filipino descent, finding a bone marrow match was really difficult. If the bone marrow match wasn't close, then it would create unbelievable suffering for Luke. The bone marrow transplant doctor confirmed that a partial match would be extremely hard on Luke and that is not what we wanted for him.

Describe how you felt at this moment, with a new baby and not only a relapse, but a terminal diagnosis?

There are no words to describe how we felt after we were told Luke was terminal. The thought of watching Luke die was overwhelming. I was angry with God and angry at the world. After Phil and I arrived home, I sat in the car by myself and screamed at God. Our faith had been shaken. I was furious that He allowed this to happen to our sweet Luke. I cried in our car by myself many times throughout Luke's ALL treatment. I was angry about Luke's situation, but also angry that Jeremy and Daniel were going to lose their brother. Phil and I pulled ourselves together and prayed and asked God to help us make the best decisions for Luke. We asked God to help Luke survive this first round of horrific chemotherapy so he could spend time with us and his brothers again.

After Luke's first round of chemotherapy for his relapse, bad things started to happen. Luke's liver was enlarged, and his stomach was bloated. Then he developed pneumonia. His oncologists told me if he didn't respond to the antibiotics and diuretics, he might have to go on a ventilator. She then said we might want to plan his funeral. I couldn't believe she actually said that, and I told her that was a horrible thing to say in front of Luke and she just walked off. Luke disliked her from the start, and I wish we had switched to a different oncologist when we first met her. Luke was very ill, so I don't think he heard what she said.

I'm still so angry about that day, that conversation…

They moved Luke into a private room, which was the best thing. Phil and I stayed with Luke during the day and took turns staying overnight with Luke during this time. I was lying there with him praying for him all night. I also asked God to help him recover from the pneumonia and to please give us more time with Luke so he could go home and see his brothers one more time. I told God that even if it was only one day at home, we would be forever grateful.

You are clearly a very faithful person and still are. Yet, you were pissed at God. How did your faith shift out of that anger?

It was at this point that I stopped being angry at God. I accepted what was happening and understood that our children truly do not belong to us, they belong to God, and we are not in control. I could tell that God blessed me with peace and understanding. Luke had gone to a few bible classes. He knew about God and liked to pray. He was a beautiful, innocent child who was going to be an angel.

The next day, God granted us a miracle. Luke's pneumonia got under control, so he didn't have to go on a ventilator. Luke had been in the hospital for a month recovering from the side effects of the horrific chemotherapy, but it got him into remission. When we took Luke home, he was happy to be home, but it was heartbreaking when he asked if he could play with his toys. It was sad because Luke had been gone for a long while, so he felt like a stranger in his own home.

It was at this point that you made a bold decision on behalf of Luke. Please tell that story.

Phil and I had long conversations about Luke's path. The oncologist said Luke needed to come back for more chemotherapy in two weeks so he would stay in remission. The thought of going back and getting more horrific chemotherapy and him possibly dying from all the side effects with an already terminal status didn't feel right.

We prayed a lot together, with our church, our family, and our friends. We accepted that Luke was terminal and wanted him to live his best life with us. I totally believed that Luke should not continue with more chemotherapy. Since Luke was terminal, I wanted Luke to enjoy his time with us and his brothers. At first, Phil had a difficult time with the decision to choose quality of life. We asked God to help us make the right decision for Luke. We had seen several cancer kids go through horrible chemotherapy to get back into remission and they died painful deaths. After a lot of prayers and discussion, we chose quality of life for Luke.

Making this choice was bold. And powerful. How did you make that happen for your child?

We met with Luke's oncologist and told her we

chose quality of life for Luke. She was shocked and asked us why we chose it. Oncologists normally don't see parents choosing quality of life, but we made the right choice for Luke with God's help. She told us that Luke's Acute Myelogenous Leukemia would relapse within three weeks, and she encouraged us to do more chemotherapy. We stood our ground and knew we had made the right decision. We went to the Day Clinic and oncology ward to say goodbye to Luke's wonderful nurses. There were a lot of tears and loving hugs, and Luke was so happy. We never told Luke he was terminal. We told him he was done with the cancer medicine and now we were going to have fun all the time.

Once that decision was made, how did your lives change?

Life felt strange after that decision, because we knew Luke was terminal, but we wanted to focus on having fun together, even though a cloud of worry hovered over us. We took Luke to Disneyland, went to visit his best friend, Alex, in Grover Beach, went fishing, and visited our families and friends. We bought the boys little battery powered ATVs and made them a path they could drive on in our yard. We took Luke to Legoland and met our longtime friend, Danielle, at Sea World and had so much fun.

Luke really loved Danielle, and they ate this big ice cream sundae together. The funniest thing was that Luke never ate much sugar, so when he ate a big part of that ice cream sundae, he was on a total sugar high. He was laughing and screaming and jumping around like a crazy person. When we put him in his car seat, he immediately fell asleep.

What did you do to keep him mentally and physically strong while terminal?

We started juicing green vegetables and apples for Luke every day. Luke loved drinking the green juice and helped put veggies in the juicer. We wanted to keep Luke as healthy as possible. His hair grew back thicker, and his skin was brighter. We would steam a bunch of broccolis, put it in a bowl, and the boys would eat it all. We looked into alternative treatments to help Luke strengthen his body and keep him healthy. We considered acupuncture and doing Rife (electromagnetic frequency). We decided we would do Rife three days a week and continue to juice every day. Luke always had a positive attitude, no matter what happened. He seemed so carefree and loved being around his family and friends.

We wanted Luke to have the experience of going to school, so we had him attend school for three months at Ms. Diana's house, where he learned his alphabet, sang, painted, and made some friends. One of Luke's friends, Nichole, who was a cancer kid at LPCH, went to this little homeschool too. We were grateful that Luke had a chance to experience school.

Years later, Luke began to decline, and the AML returned. When it was clear he was passing away, how did you decide on a meaningful way to honor him, and how did you ultimately bid him farewell?

Twenty-seven months after his last chemo, Luke's Acute Myelogenous Leukemia returned. It was incredible that God gave us twenty-seven months with Luke instead of the three weeks the oncologist predicted. We knew Luke's time was running out, but we just didn't know when. It was overwhelming and heartbreaking to know we had to say goodbye to Luke soon. Phil and I were deeply saddened and stressed because we knew time was running out for Luke. This kind of situation creates so much intense anxiety and grief. Phil and I comforted each other and asked God to help us survive saying goodbye to Luke.

In the last two months of Luke's life, he had a couple of blood transfusions. We knew it was time to let him go to heaven. We called our family and friends, and they all came to give Luke a hug and kiss goodbye. Phil's brothers and their wives, Bob and Julie, and Larry and Carol, flew in from Los Angeles and Santa Fe. Our family sang songs for Luke, and we know he felt the love. Jeremy and Daniel kissed Luke goodbye and laid with Luke in his bed. We had our family drop Jeremy and Daniel off at our house with a babysitter so we could say our goodbyes to Luke.

Arne and I were there. And I have never seen such a thoughtful, beautiful goodbye day. You created a room that was filled with light, love, tenderness, music, and positive energy for Luke to feel safe to depart. And for you to feel safe to let him, I'd imagine . . .

After our family and friends left the hospital, we talked to Luke and told him it was okay to leave and go to the light. We told him we would be okay and that he would be with us in spirit, and he could see us anytime. We promised Luke we would take care of Jeremy and Daniel and that we would have as much fun as possible in honor of him. There are no words to describe saying your final goodbyes to your child. We held him close, kissed him when he took his last breath, and asked God to help us in this truly devastating moment. The thought of leaving him in that hospital room was so difficult for both of us. How could we walk out of his hospital room and leave him there? Luke died on August 11, 2001, at 4pm. We stayed with him for as long as we could and then went home. We were relieved he wasn't suffering anymore, but our hearts were shattered.

How did you tell the kids? What advice do you have for other parents in this situation?

Phil and I decided not to tell Jeremy and Daniel that Luke had died. We were in bad shape, completely mentally and emotionally distraught, and couldn't talk about it. We gave Jeremy and Daniel a bath and we all slept in our bed together. Jeremy slept next to me and that was such a comfort. At one o'clock in the morning, Jeremy started to laugh out loud and kick his feet, so it woke me up. I kissed Jeremy and told him he needed to go to sleep. Jeremy kept laughing and kicking his feet until five o'clock in the morning. I was so exhausted. I told Jeremy to please go to sleep. Jeremy said, "Mom, could you please tell Luke to stop tickling me?" I was in tears because I knew Luke was tickling Jeremy and he came to visit us, letting us know he was okay.

I told Luke we had to get some sleep so could he please stop tickling Jeremy. Suddenly, I felt warmth and tingling in both my cheeks and on my arm. It was Luke. He was giving me a kiss and a hug. I just lay there and felt his love. I was so incredibly grateful because he truly was free and saying hello to us.

The next day, Phil and I told Jeremy that Luke had died. Jeremy was four years old, and Daniel was two years old when Luke died. Jeremy cried hard when we told him that Luke died. Luke and Jeremy were very close, and Jeremy was mad that Luke didn't tell him he was going to die. We explained to Jeremy that it wasn't Luke's fault, and that God needed Luke to be an angel in heaven and that we would see Luke again. Jeremy cried with us, and we all grieved together. Daniel didn't really understand what was going on.

Jeremy wanted to see Luke, so we played our family video with Luke that we had made six months earlier. We all sat down in our living room and watched the video. We were all crying and suddenly we heard Luke's favorite dinosaur roaring from Luke's bedroom. The crazy thing was that Luke always complained that the button on that dinosaur was always hard to push, which made the roaring even more special. We were so grateful that Luke came to visit again.

In the aftermath of Luke's passing, how did you and your family find solace and honor his memory as you lived with the loss and heartache?

Luke's memorial service and funeral were really hard on us. We were relieved when it was over. We were grateful to all the people who came to honor Luke, but we were mentally and emotionally exhausted. A month later, the Leukemia Society South Bay running group held a tree planting ceremony in honor of Luke and his birthday. It was a beautiful way to celebrate Luke's birthday.

The Leukemia Society South Bay Running Group

wanted to continue to have a Luke's Run as a
fundraising event and to celebrate Luke's birthday.
We were grateful. We continued Luke's Run for
seven years.

This was a MASSIVE annual party that brought so much good to the world. This was an incredible gift to the community, and it meant a lot to our entire family to participate in Luke's Run.

Two months later, I wasn't doing well without Luke.
I was missing him terribly and wanted to talk to
him. Phil wasn't doing well either, but men tend to
hide their grief better than women. I cried every
day and wasn't sure how I was going to make it,
especially having to take care of a two- and a four-
year-old. Jeremy asked me how long I was going
to cry, and I told him it would probably be a long
time. We kept the kids busy, and we put Jeremy in
preschool.

Do you recommend grief therapy? What impact did it have on your family?

We put Jeremy in a grief group with other kids, and
it was good for him. He was having anxiety issues
about Luke's passing and was dealing with a lot of
grief.

We met other nice parents who had lost children.
Phil and I also went to grief therapy. It was helpful
to talk about how we were coping.

It was really tough meeting these parents in this
grief group and knowing how their children died.
Some of their children had died in car accidents, or
from illnesses or homicides. It really opened our eyes
to a whole other world of loss. After three months

of once-a-week grief therapy, Jeremy asked to stop going to it. He said it was good for him, but it was making him sad. Grief therapy is helpful, but I can see how it can be tough finding out about how all these children died.

And, bottom line, you simply missed your baby. I know that something very magical happened to you during this time—and it happened because you advocated for yourself and what you needed. Please tell us.

During this time, I was doing my best to help a couple of other parents whose kids were still battling cancer. I brought food to some families at the hospital, and we donated to their family funds. It was therapy for me to give back because I knew what that life was like. After their kids left the hospital or passed away, we still donated toys to the Day Clinic's treasure box. Luke always loved going to the treasure box after getting a shot.

I never thought I would be so depressed that I would think about suicide. I didn't think I would do it, but I could see how depression could put me in such a bad place. I wanted to be able to talk to Luke. Phil and I prayed and asked God to help heal our hearts and our hopelessness. It was like we were lost. Through a distant contact, I found a psychic. I called her up and convinced Phil that we needed to see if we could talk to Luke. Phil was skeptical, and I understood his perspective, but I told him I really needed to make sure Luke was okay.

This psychic was from the east coast and would do readings in the Bay Area every three to six months. She knew nothing about Luke and our family. I didn't even give her our last name when I made the appointment. When our meeting with the psychic started, she prayed and asked God for protection for all of us and that only positive information be passed on. Immediately afterwards, she said that there was a little boy wanting to talk to us. She said he was smiling and waving something yellow. Phil and I both broke down in tears because we knew he was telling us it was him.

The yellow thing he was waving was his favorite yellow blanket that our friend Polly had made for him. Only our family and close friends knew about the significance of that yellow blanket.

She told us that Luke said he loved us very much and that he did not want us to cry so much for him because he was always with us. He said he was happy, and God had him welcoming other children into heaven. She told us he was holding something, and it looked like a frog. Jeremy's frog had died the day before our meeting with the psychic and when we buried it, Jeremy asked Luke to please take care of his frog. Again, it confirmed for us that Luke was with us, which was so heartwarming. We asked the crazy question about why this happened to Luke. She told us that before any of us are born we have an agreement with God about what will happen in our lives. Apparently, Luke agreed and spiritually knew he would suffer through cancer treatment and die at six years old. It was all part of his life lesson, and he had to learn from it.

All of us parents who have lost a loved one, dealt with a chronic illness, terrible hardship, or a death of their child always ask that "why" question. No matter what religion we are part of, no one can give a good answer, but the psychic's answer made more sense and helped us with acceptance.

How is your family healing now, over twenty years later? What promises did you and Phil make to each other about living life without Luke?

Phil and I were lucky that we could work together well as a team throughout Luke's journey. I am fortunate to have a husband who is incredibly supportive, kind, always willing to help and to work things out. This journey of trying to save Luke was full of emotional, physical, and mental stress. The grief lingers. While Jeremy and Daniel were growing up, they had all these fun experiences and milestones. At every fun experience, birthday, or success, we always think about Luke and what could have been. Phil and I did not tell the boys, but the first thing we think of whenever they have something to celebrate is Luke. We also continue to thank God that he gave us an extra twenty-seven months with Luke. We will forever be grateful to God for that because we know that is a rare gift.

We had promised Luke that we would make Jeremy and Daniel's life fun and happy, no matter what. We bought a home on a local river that has a dock, and the boys have grown up fishing, kayaking, jet skiing, and boating. We throw rose petals in the river in honor of Luke's birthday every year and he is still a big part of our lives wherever we go.

Luke's best friend, Alex, who is now thirty years old, is doing great. We absolutely love him and his parents, Jeniene and Jeff. We have stayed close, and we are so proud of Alex. Every time we see Alex, it is emotional because he fought his battle with cancer and survived. Seeing him reminds us of Luke, but it is a positive and loving experience. We received Alex and Tad's 2023 wedding invitation, and we were shocked at the date of their wedding. They had no idea their wedding was on Luke's birthday. We thanked Luke because we know he had a part in helping them pick his birthday as their wedding date. On the day of their wedding, we arrived at the hotel and one of our favorite family songs with Luke, Ain't No Mountain High Enough, started playing in the lobby as we entered. We started singing it and knew our angel Luke was there with us.

He was letting you know, yet again, "I'm right here with you!"

It can be a gray area believing in whether our loved ones can communicate with us after they pass away. We have been lucky enough that God allowed us to talk to Luke through a psychic and also have him visit us. Having faith in God during this journey of battling cancer or any other life-threatening illness is important. Even if we all have different religious beliefs, faith can give you courage, which helps you face what scares you and gives you strength in the face of grief or pain.

16

Grandparents, Friends & Family

The smallest act of kindness is worth more than the greatest intention.

KHALIL GIBRAN

Your best friend, coworker, daughter, or cousin just got slammed with the worst news—their child has cancer. You are spiraling with love, concern, and are completely paralyzed. Sound familiar? No judgment here. We've all been there. Even those of us who've walked down the dark road of childhood cancer fall into that paralysis trap when another friend is suffering. It happens.

But we can do better.

This chapter is specifically for parents, grandparents, friends, coworkers, and family. It's designed to give you a place to get helpful and brutally honest advice not only from me, but from current parents in the trenches of cancer treatment as of 2024. Their quotes, along with tips and tricks that are proven to help relieve the stress on your person in crisis, will hopefully bring you closer together during this trying time, instead of pulling you apart. For ease, I'm going to refer to the best friend/coworker/daughter/cousin as your "person."

A Special Note For Grandparents

Dear grandparents, what a tough situation you are in right now. My heart goes out to you as you grieve and are filled with worry and despair for both your child and grandchild. This stressful situation can bring out the best and the worst in an existing parent-child relationship. Tempers flare, misunderstandings abound, and yet beneath it all is great love. While this entire chapter (and this entire book) will be of enormous help to you, here are some tips and tricks just for you.

> *Grandparents have to understand that sometimes they won't have free access to their grandbaby like they once had. When counts are low, medication regiments are complicated, etc., they need to try not to take it personally when we keep everyone, including them, away.* —**ANONYMOUS**

💡 Toolbox Tip:

- Be present. Be present without judgment, just love.

- Let your child take the lead and follow their example.

- Monitor your emotions. Of course, you are devastated but losing it in front of your child (or grandchild) regularly isn't helpful as it just gives them one more thing to worry about—you. Certainly, feel all the feelings—just do it privately.

- Show your love with actions: For example, hire a cleaning service to come once a week. Kids on chemo should avoid germs because their immune systems are compromised.

- Your child and grandchild will be spending an inpatient month in the hospital (called "in-patient"). If you live far away and can swing it, move in or nearby for the first month.

- Water the plants, tidy up, take Fido for a daily walk, stock the fridge, buy flowers.

- FaceTime or call as often as the parents are comfortable but be understanding and gracious if they don't answer every time.

Check in with your kiddo/cancer kid parent, too, because they likely miss you just as much as your grandchild. Just tell them how proud you are of how well they're facing this battle and helping their child fight.

- If you live nearby, volunteer to do a regular chore or errands for the next several months until the family gets their bearings: grocery shopping, watering of plants, taking care of deliveries.

Anything and everything helps. I'll never forget the simple act of my mom hearing me complain about how cold I was at the hospital and how she showed up a few hours later with a cozy new sweatshirt and sweatpants.

My mom was our biggest help! She is retired and would come to stay with us for months. She would watch our non-CK (cancer kid) while we did hospital stays and treatments. When we did one week hospital stays for chemo, on Thursday she and our non-CK kid would come to visit, and we would play games for a few hours and then Mom would decorate the door differently every time we came home.

When school started, I wanted my non-cancer child to start back at school so we moved in with Mom so she would watch my CK. My mom is a retired teacher and gave daily lessons to my girl.

There is NO way we could have taken on the world of cancer alone.

My mother-in-law, who is not retired, would come every two weeks and bring us bulk necessities and visit our kids. She would stay weekends when my CK had high counts and would spend the

day painting, having tea parties, and loving on the girls so we
could get out. Showing up when able and taking the deep dive
with us was a huge blessing in our journey. **—ANONYMOUS**

My parents, Pauline and Glenn, truly kicked into gear when they found their calling as our helpers. They became The Hospital Party Planners. I don't remember if I asked them to create The Hospital Party or if they volunteered, but boy once they were on board, did they own it. That was their calling (see Chapter 9 for details). My mother-in-law, Marie, had been a professional nanny as a young woman, so she and my father-in-law, Nils, naturally gravitated towards taking care of Madi's needs. That was their calling. Find your calling, the thing that helps the most and plays to your strengths.

The rest of this chapter is designed for all friends, family, and grandparents. Let's get to it.

Friends and Family: Step Up and Pitch In

"Let me know what I can do for you!" is a well-intentioned phrase that all of us have been guilty of saying. A cancer parent is on overload, and they don't have the capacity to figure out what they need and then tell you. So, look around, listen, be observant, play to your strengths and take action.

Are you a magnificent organizer? Volunteer to be their Point Person and recruit your friend community to help. Love to cook? Show up with dinner every Friday. Are you a great gardener? Come twice a week to water and tend to their indoor and outdoor flowers. Get the drift? If you are living far from your person, know that there is so much you can do and organize from a distance. Check out Chapter 6 and the Toolbox Tips at the end of this chapter for a full list of ideas for those near and far.

The people who felt the most helpful to me were the ones who
didn't ask what I needed. The people who did whatever they could
think of, regardless if it was the "right" thing. People brought us
care packages and planted flowers so I could see them bloom
when I had no energy to put into my yard. A friend baked us

sourdough bread regularly because it was one of the only foods that tasted good to my son even when he was nauseated. None of these people put it on me to figure out what I needed. I now know that when people are walking through crisis, any little bit of showing them that you're trying to help carry the load with them matters. It doesn't matter what's in the care package or the groceries or the card. It matters that they tried and that they love you. **—ANNA**

💡 Toolbox Tip:

Instead of asking "how can I help", say "I'm bringing dinner over next Tuesday. Do you prefer chicken or burgers?" Or "I'm coming over Monday between one and three to hang out with your kids. Plan to take a nap or a walk." Not giving your person an option to say no is the best choice for successfully helping them.

Plenty of people have said, "Let me know if you need anything." While the intentions are good, it's too hard to ask for help. I have a few friends who just told me what they were going to do. "We're planning some meals for you. Any preferences or dislikes?" I'd recommend people make a concrete offer of help, something specific, then it's so much easier to accept. **—KATRINA**

Help by stopping in and just visiting and distracting the kids so (parents) can breathe regularly—and help with the things you know they struggle with, without asking. Asking for help constantly can feel defeating. **—VICTORIA MARIE**

Don't Go Turtle

It's a common mistake: You don't know what to do, so instead of reaching out, you turtle (tuck in and hide), with some excuse such as, "I thought you needed your space." And if we are being honest with ourselves, that's a cop out. When we turtle, we make the situation about us—our discomfort, fear, and anxiety. It's a well-known fact in the childhood cancer world that a cancer diagnosis makes friends disappear. People fear the word cancer and run. You truly find out who your people are when you are in a crisis. Rise above your fear and talk to your person. Often. Even if they don't respond, keep reaching out.

> I would encourage friends and family to continue to reach out. Sometimes it feels like you are forgotten. I'm sure a lot of it is that people don't know what to say but saying nothing almost feels worse. I can't even tell you how many friends seemed to disappear throughout our journey, and it feels pretty crappy. This journey feels so isolating in general, so feeling forgotten on top of that really hurts. —**ANONYMOUS**

> Ask how things are going. So many people are afraid to ask. They don't want to impose; they don't want to bring it up in case we don't want to talk about it. But leave that up to us. Ask. Let us know you care. If you don't ask, we think you don't care. —**SONIA**

Your person isn't the same right now. They probably aren't communicating normally or telling you what they want and need. They might be snippy, tearful, raging, or silent. All of those reactions are normal. Having a child diagnosed with a life-threatening disease throws you into the trenches so fast and the job is so huge that you don't have time to focus on anything but helping your kid to survive. Know this and set a reminder to reach out often. This is especially true if their child relapses or worse, dies. Never abandon them, no matter what. Commit to travelling with them wherever this journey leads and let them know you'll always be by their side.

Don't Take No For An Answer

It's common for a parent of a kid with cancer, when asked what they need or if they would like dinner delivered, to say, "No, that's okay." They don't mean it. We live in a society that is terrible about asking for help, so that phrase "No, that's okay", comes flying out of our mouths without much thought. We don't want to impose, which is ridiculous and completely unhelpful. So don't take no for an answer. Of course, be respectful, but stick with it. Offer the help, dinner, or childcare by setting a date and not giving them the option of "no." Instead, say, "I'm sending a cleaning service to your house next Friday at 10am. It's all paid for." Nobody is going to say no to that!

> When we first got back from the hospital, I was in a fog, depressed, scared, and in total momma-bear mood. I didn't want to leave the house or leave my child because I learned first-hand that things change from one minute to the next. I was invited out for a quick lunch by the aunts, and I said no. I couldn't and didn't want to leave. What would I say? How would they react if I just broke down (which I totally did)? How could I leave? What if something happened? They did not take no for an answer. They came over, waited outside for me, and took me to lunch. It was the breath of fresh air I didn't know I needed.
>
> I NEEDED to step away and be reminded that while this IS hard and it IS brutal, you can still find peace in the little moments, and life won't always be dark. You NEED to get your cup filled so you can continue to pour. It was my first time thinking, "Ok, we can do this." We cried, we laughed, we sat in silence, and then slowly it was like the cloud lifted . . . just for a little bit . . . it gave me the strength I needed to come back and pour some of that strength and positivity back into my home. **—AUDREY**
>
> . . . don't take "no" for an answer to "how can I help?" **—VICTORIA**
>
> Visit—sit and talk. Bring some dinner, or even better, a couple of margaritas. **—ALYSSA**

Remember The Siblings

> Don't forget about the siblings. They are the forgotten heroes. Often feeling left out, scared, they may have resentment. Ask them how they are doing, not just how their sibling with cancer is doing. **—SONIA**

This topic is so important that I've devoted much of Chapter 12 to the needs of siblings. During our first month of treatment, many well-meaning colleagues and friends came bearing gifts for Cecilia—too many! Thankfully, the girls were not around when two huge toy baskets came to the house, and in a rare moment of clarity, I shoved them deep into the closet. This way we could take control of when the kids needed a new little something during a tough day, or a long hospital stay.

Friends, family, and grandparents: Don't shy away from bringing over a treasure but be sure to include the whole family. Maybe it's a new game they can all play, or a different toy for each child. Just remember to acknowledge them, too, in words and deeds. They are also suffering and can feel very left out in this process if all the focus and attention goes to their sibling with cancer.

Cancer Is A Marathon—Stay in the Race

Childhood cancer often comes with lengthy treatments, often years long. At some point, parents may attempt to make life appear normal, either for their own sanity, or their children's mental health. But that does not mean they are feeling normal on the inside. Childhood cancer is an insidious visitor, and it's not until your child is well past the five-year mark that you stop looking over your shoulder in fear of relapse and start to truly exhale. Remember that and set yourself a reminder to regularly check in with your person. If you know a hospital stay or check-up is imminent, even if it's expected and two years into treatment, do something kind for your person: Have coffee delivered; DoorDash a delicious healthy lunch; swing by and offer to read their kid a book while they go for a walk around the block. It means the world to have that support for the duration because this lengthy cancer marathon is lonely.

> My granddaughter was fourteen months old when she was
> first diagnosed with Acute Lymphoblastic Leukemia in 2018.
> Comments such as, "At least she's young enough she won't
> remember" aren't true or helpful. Our bodies remember and

*whether or not she fully remembers, the trauma is there. She
finished treatment in February 2021, and we were so excited
to celebrate her "five years cured" in 2023. Instead, she
ended up being part of the four in one million kids to develop
Myelodysplastic Syndrome, MDS for short. MDS is its own cancer
and a precursor to AML. This is a direct result of the chemo
used to treat her leukemia from 2018-2021. She turned seven
yesterday and has undergone a stem cell transplant thanks to
her perfect match, her three-year-old little sister. She's doing
great and is currently cancer-free.* **—JENNY L.**

*A reminder to check in and care six months or more down the
road. I felt like everyone wanted to help during that first month
of diagnosis and when we were in-patient and then after that it
dropped off, outside of wanting updates. It felt like no one cared
any longer.* **—ALICIA**

What Not To Say

There are a few things that universally drive a cancer parent up the
wall or brings them to tears. And unless you have gone through
something similar, you wouldn't know! So, let me help you with
Toolbox Tips of "Things never to say to a cancer parent." Or,
really, anybody going through something hard.

⊘ "I don't know how you do it."

Oh, we heard this often. Listen up. Nobody signs up for parenting a
kid with cancer. And we didn't get the job because we can "handle
it." I'm not stronger than you, shit just happens and it happens to
all of us.

*One of my biggest 'don't say that' is "You're so much stronger than
I am; I couldn't do this." It's not helpful and is almost dismissive.
Everyone would opt out if they had the option. We don't have the
option, so shut up. It's not encouraging at all!* **—ALICIA**

⊘ **"God needs another angel" or "God is so cruel to do this to a child."**

Bullshit. Utter nonsense. Dig into any faith practice and you will find that God, Buddha, Bhagavan, or the Universe are all about love, light, and hope. They are who people go to for strength.

No faith practice has a God who punishes small children and their parents by giving kids cancer.

Just stop.

⊘ **"My son is sick and I'm so worried. How was your child diagnosed?"**

This was said to me… more than once. Do not equate your child's cold or fever with cancer. Yes, it can be scary when your child is sick, especially when you are watching one of all of our biggest fears come to life in front of your eyes! But your kid does not have cancer. If need be, share your fears with your doctor, not the parent of the child with cancer. It's annoying.

I also heard, "Oh, a friend of a friend also had cancer, and they died." I couldn't believe people said this to me! In retrospect, I think they were looking for any experience they could relate to my own. This is not necessary. I think a lot of people's first reaction is to try to relate, but it often does more harm than good.
—BROOK, AML/BMT SURVIVOR; MEDICAL STUDENT

⊘ **"I can't come to the hospital to visit again. It was just too hard."**

And sadly, this too was actually said to me. I have one reaction to that: **Really? Hard for YOU?**

If you are freaked out by the yellow bags of biohazard and needles, so is your person. Either take a deeper breath and don't make it about you or find another way to help without telling your person the hospital was "too hard."

⊘ **"How are you doing, sweetie? You don't look sick!"**

Please don't refer to a kid fighting cancer as "sick." If your person's child has hit remission, they are "in treatment." Big difference.

As an educator with over thirty years of experience, I know first-hand that words matter to children. They absorb everything. If people around them continually tell them they are sick, fragile, weak, they will believe it. I've watched this happen and have seen children shrink, wither, and stop fighting under the pressure of those kinds of insidious words—which is the last thing you want, right?

You want them to feel strong, healthy, and normal even if they are in treatment for cancer. Lift them up with positive language.

Top Things A Cancer Parent Needs

Okay, you've heard my advice and now it's time to get going and help! Everybody loves a to-do list, especially when it's been curated and designed to help your person feel better. Some ideas are free, others take some time or money. Pick what you can manage and go for it!

Volunteer To Be The Point Person

If you are great with a spreadsheet and organizing people, within the first two weeks let your person know you'll be their Point Person. You should know your person well enough for them to feel comfortable being honest with you about what they need and with letting you take control. Just remember, "What do you need?" isn't a helpful question. Instead, let your person know you will be organizing friends and family to help with these items: meals, home care, babysitting, etc.—whatever you know your person needs because you know them well and you observe their everyday needs (childcare) and wants (a massage). You might be their best friend, treasured cousin, or a buddy from work. This job can be done whether you're nearby or far away.

Remember this—people LOVE a job and generally, want to help. Develop a shared Google Doc that itemizes what your person needs and when and send it out once a week early on, monthly later. Remember to add all those little errands that need to be done—pick up the dry cleaning, drop off a package, take your youngest to and from dance class, etc.

> ## Toolbox Tip:
> People will sometimes offer to pay for those groceries and errands. Let them.

Meal Prep

Assign one friend or a family member to set up your food requests on a site like mealtrain.com, where you can specify the family's wishes for meals and the appropriate days and times for delivery. Consider having dinners delivered for the first month or two of treatment while families get their bearings, and a couple of times a month thereafter. This can be a separate job from those given to the Point Person, or the Point Person could simply provide a link to Meal Train to get that going.

> ## Toolbox Tip:
> Set up a large cooler outside your person's front door for meal deliveries. They may want to chat, they may not, or they might be at the hospital. A cooler gives them options.

Updates

Everybody wants an update, and talking on the phone or sharing on social media might be way too much to handle during treatment, especially in the beginning. But that's when everybody wants details! Are you technically skilled and a good writer? Offer to set up a way to share information with friends and family.

> ## Toolbox Tip:
> You can set up a sharing site in a variety of ways, from creating a Facebook page to using the popular CaringBridge website at www.caringbridge.org where either you, or your person, can provide updates as desired.

Help During Hospital Stays

Some hospital stays are a planned part of treatment, and others are a total surprise. My daughter's cancer, ALL, had six planned hospital stays for more intensive chemo that had to be monitored more closely. And a fever will always mean a trip to the hospital for observation and possible intervention because a child's immune system is low, and they may need help fighting an infection. If your person's child is inpatient and stable, you will need some boredom relief while you endure their stay. (See The Hospital Party chapter for ideas for planned stays.)

Visits break up the day for parents and are something to look forward to. But showing up at the hospital, especially if you are not used to seeing kids hooked up to an IV with a yellow bag labeled "biohazard", can feel scary if you aren't mentally prepared. A visit might be delivering a favorite coffee to your person before you head to work, dropping off dinner, or doing a puzzle with their child while you send your person outside to walk around the block in the sun and breathe. Mentally prepare your mood before you arrive and bring only lightness and love to a visit, not fear and tears.

Your person might be reluctant to leave their kid, so confidently show them you've got it for thirty minutes and send them outside. Or, if you are close to the child, come by for a movie afternoon and let your friend go nap, hit the chapel, wander the mall, get a massage. (Book that massage for them and, if you can, pay for it in advance—what a treat!).

Remember, if hospitals and sick children are going to freak you out to the point that it's all about you, do something else to help. Your person needs people to visit who can "bring the party" in terms of attitude and fun. It's your job to help them feel better about their situation and to lift them up, not the other way around!

Note: If you are a best friend, sibling, or a grandparent and you are terrified of the hospital, I get it. You still need to be there, so get some therapy, take a deep breath, or journal about your feelings and go. A best friend or grandparent not showing up will have severe consequences on the relationship. They need you.

> ## Toolbox Tip:
>
> When we were in-patient and stable, a bestie, Nikki, and her family would make a point to come once a week with takeout and a game.
>
> She never asked me what we wanted for dinner (she knew my preferences) or what we wanted to play—she just took charge.
>
> We would leave the hospital room, dragging the IV pole of chemo with us, and have picnic dinners in a quiet, sunny public alcove. On other days, Nikki would bring Cecilia's bestie, Tegan, to the hospital. Tegan quickly became comfortable with all the IV poles—all she saw was her buddy! They would hit the preschool playground together, or the art room, or simply lay on the bed together and watch *Teletubbies*. Nikki and I could sneak to the other side of the room or just go outside and talk. Pure gold.

You might think your child will be freaked out by seeing their friend in the hospital, but we never found that to be true. Kids are resilient and it's much scarier to imagine what's going on with their little friend than it is to actually see them.

Getting out of a hospital room, when allowed, will completely change your person's mindset, and offer some fun and normalcy to the day.

A Special Treat

My parents taught me that it's the little things in life that really brighten your day. Fresh flowers from the garden in the kitchen, a lovely cup of tea, or playing music you love can change your outlook. During this marathon, what would be a special treat for your person? What do they need help with mentally and physically? Parents often forget to ask for help for themselves, but everybody needs a special treat.

> ## Toolbox Tip:
>
> • Have a group of friends or colleagues book a massage package.
>
> • Order flowers or fresh fruit to be delivered once a month.

- Take your friend out for a mani-pedi.

- Offer to come every Thursday so the parent(s) or partners can go out to dinner.

- Stop by randomly with a favorite coffee or tea, and fold that pile of laundry on the sofa while you gab.

- Create a kick-ass playlist on Spotify to inspire them.

- Send them a cool meditation link they'd enjoy.

- Buy tickets to that movie they wanted to see (with babysitting included).

- Take them to their favorite workout class or a day pass at a fancy gym and sweat it out.

A special treat is very personal. So, think about what your person loves, and make it happen for them.

Keep Them Healthy

If you are local and part of the family's inner circle socially or at school, one big way you can help is to do your best to keep the child in treatment healthy. Chemo tanks immune systems and makes a child vulnerable to scary illnesses, illnesses that can harm them faster than cancer. Be vigilant, practical, and communicate with your person before playdates and birthday parties. Calmly be the watchdog for your friend group and call out anybody who isn't being responsible for the health of all (preferably without your person knowing). This should be fairly easy after COVID-19 as most of us got incredibly good about taking care of each other and not exposing anyone to unnecessary germs.

♀ Toolbox Tip:

- If you have a playdate planned and either you or your child wakes up with the sniffles, cancel calmly with love. Set up the next one for a week later.

- When you arrive for a playdate, get into the habit of squirting your hand and your kid's hand with hand sanitizer and/or just wash up for thirty or so seconds.

- If you are giving your person a break and hosting the kids at your house, don't worry about letting them go crazy. Let them make a mess and get dirty. Just regularly squirt that hand sanitizer and/or wash up without making a big deal about it, and certainly without saying, "Well you need to honey, because you have cancer." (Yes, this happened to Cecilia).

- Remove shoes before entering the house. Shoes track in an enormous amount of germs from the outside world that may pose health risks to the child in treatment.

- If you are at the end of a cold, mask up if you are in a social setting with the family, just in case.

You Are a Gift

I hope this chapter has given you clarity and specific ideas for how to help a family in crisis. Too many of us fly blind and are terrified when our co-workers, friends, and family members are sick and in despair and it's especially awful when it's someone's kid. We want to help; we just don't know how. Toolbox Tips from this chapter hold everything you need to make a difference in their long cancer journey.

It's easier to care for your person and their child when things are going well. But remember, they need you at all times. Being there is crucial, especially if their child has a scary secondary illness, relapses or worse, dies.

As their person, you will suffer with grief and despair for both your person and their child, even if the outcome is positive. Stay present, get help for processing your emotions, and keep the focus on them. Commit to travelling with your person wherever this journey leads them and let them know you'll always be by their side. Thank you for reading this chapter. You are a gift to your person.

Being there means you care, and care deeply about your best

friend, coworker, child, or other relative. They will never forget your kindness.

17

Turning The Page
Creating Your Next Chapter

There are far better things ahead than
any we leave behind.

C.S. LEWIS

Toward the end of treatment, I was having coffee with a friend, looking back at the horrific battle that seemed to be almost behind us while, at the same time, trying to glimpse my future. I was spiraling on that particular day, and the "what-ifs" were taking over any vision of a positive future.

What if she relapses?

What if she really can't do math in third grade?

What if she gets sick and can't recover because her immune system is trashed?

Being a cancer parent is a full-time job, and oddly, at the end, it's a little weird to give up the role you have invested so much time, energy, and utter devotion to. As I continued to pour over future what-ifs and how I could go to battle with all of them (as we cancer parents tend to do), my friend looked at me and said, "You know, what if you tried to look at this whole experience as just a chapter in your lives, instead of the whole story?"

Wow. Hearing that from a treasured friend who witnessed it all made me realize the truth: It was up to us to write the rest of our story. It's a choice to move on and create the next chapter of your life after cancer, and to not continuously stress about what might happen. If you don't make that leap of faith, you risk being that parent who continually talks about and lives with cancer long after the scary part is over. I didn't want to be that mom. I bet you don't want to be that parent either.

My conversation with that friend reminded me of a story from the beginning of our journey.

Right after the Consolidation phase of our treatment (at about six months), our amazing nurse practitioner, Stacey, gently nudged us to try living more normally. To have some fun. She always made even the hardest days fun for Cecilia, with her big smile and positive outlook. She told us about an incredible camp for kids with cancer and their families—Camp Okizu. Like many camps for kids with cancer, Camp Okizu was loaded with fun for the kids in a safe environment where nurses were on hand to administer chemo and keep a watchful eye as the kids went crazy. Stacey told us that families had a chance to rest and restore, and parents would have the opportunity to gather and participate in a guided talk. THIS is what I was most excited about. Help! People who had "been there, done that" and could offer their sage advice and provide cheerleading. I was pumped.

For Cecilia, the weekend at Camp Okizu was magical. Incredible camp organizers and counselors meticulously planned abundant camp activities and all forms of fun and games.

The entire program was overseen by doctors and nurses who volunteered their time to make sure the children were safe, and that treatment could continue while the fun ensued. Cecilia made friends, saw children who got pokes like her, and, most importantly, she could just be a kid. She relished the camp counselor's attention, made friendship bracelets galore, swam, was the top lizard-catcher of the weekend, and was head-to-toe filthy every day. It was awesome. (See Resources for camps near you.)

But what unfolded on that cloudy spring afternoon at Camp Okizu for us in the parent meeting was quite different. It became what shaped the entire rest of our journey.

Moderators gently asked the group how they were doing and what strategies they were using to cope. Answers began flowing easily . . . but not in the form of advice or from a place of wisdom. The entire ninety minutes was spent in a place of despair. The parents in attendance were six months, two years, ten years ahead of us in treatment. All of their kids were doing well, and many had completed treatment years prior. But they still lived with cancer at the forefront—as the main character in their story.

We raised our hands a few times to share the small but mighty coping strategies we were exploring as newbies. However, we quickly realized that as the "young'uns" in the group, it really was not our time to share wisdom. So, we listened.

By the end of those ninety minutes of tears, despair, what-ifs, grieving over lost time, and sharing stories about their child's massive side effects, I felt as though I'd had the Positude bludgeoned out of me. Of course, it was just this particular group of parents, on this particular day, who turned the conversation so negative. But the experience stuck with me.

One thing was crystal clear by the time camp ended: whatever happened, I refused to go through this and end up on the other side worse than when we started. And that conversation with my friend brought our camp experience back to the forefront of my mind. I had to make a choice that day over coffee. And I chose life and moving forward, and I choose it to this day, even when things get rough.

Years later, I'm grateful that Cecilia was blessed with the full

Camp Okizu experience. I'm also grateful for what went down for us as parents that particular weekend. That experience, as difficult as it was, became the catalyst for developing our Positude, establishing a new normal, and for paying attention to our family and *ourselves* so we wouldn't end up as another statistic. I was determined not to let that happen to me or any other cancer parent.

Creating your next chapter may seem like a lofty goal right now. The trick is, ironically, not to worry about the finish line or even about next week. Keep it simple. Make it a daily practice to focus on what's going on right now with intention and attention.

There is a lot of talk in the media about intention-setting and living with purpose. That can feel petty when your energy has been consumed by life-or-death battles like cancer survival. So, keep it real and remember how we've framed coping techniques in *The Cancer Parent's Handbook*:

- Surrender to what is. Your child has cancer and is in treatment. That is just a fact.

- Surrendering isn't giving up; it's the first step in finding your power. Accepting and surrendering to your situation, you will stop rebelling against the world. When you do that, your mind is free to problem-solve and to set clear, positive intentions for action.

- Each day, set your intention to truly see the precious small joys and treasures surrounding you. Appreciate them with gratitude, especially on the dark days.

- Choose kindness, and pause before snapping at your child, partner, oncologist, or the unsuspecting person in line at the store. Breathe.

- Normalize this experience. Do the work that needs to be done (poke, radiation, etc.) and move on.

- Make fun and play a part of everyday life so your kid can be a kid.

- Educate yourself so you can have relevant, meaningful conversations with your medical team and know when to advocate for your child and yourself.

- Ask for help. Do so boldly and without guilt.

- Pay it forward. Focusing on bringing good into the world, even when your own life is challenging, can help you get out of your negative or anxiety-filled head space.

- Restore your body, mind, and soul so you can be the warrior and advocate for your kid that you aspire to be. Make it a priority.

When you are in the middle of trauma, if you can choose to manage your situation through the lens of surrender, action, intention, play, and Positude, you will develop skills that will last a lifetime. For me, the biggest skill I found was resiliency.

Resiliency

Noun: The capacity to withstand or to recover quickly from difficulties; toughness.

Resiliency lessons from my cancer years have stuck with me and continue to inform my actions in big and small crises that come up in life. And I'm grateful! When you learn how to rise through resilience, you view trauma, setbacks, and life's inevitable challenges with an entirely new frame of mind. You find your power.

For me, resiliency isn't about hunkering down, toughing it out, waiting for the storm to pass. It's about finding creative ways to adapt to a changing landscape and riding the wave while you continue to make magic in your life. Tough times can be a huge opportunity to step back, look at the situation, find your Positude and resiliency, and not just survive but thrive. Yes, thrive. Even through the fire.

The decision to live with a positive outlook, to see the good in each day and the joy in front of you makes an enormous difference in your entire family's mental and physical outcome during a cancer journey. I'm sure of it. Try something positive today. Start that nightly gratitude journal. Have a morning meditation before everyone in the house wakes up. And every day, find the good that's still in life and let it be a source of comfort and strength on difficult days.

★ ★ ★

You've got this.

I hope *The Cancer Parent's Handbook* will remain by your bedside or on your kitchen table so you can read and re-read it as often as you need to in order to be lifted up and reminded that you have a voice, options, and a massive toolbox now at your disposal. May it be dog-eared and highlighted as you craft your way of existing within the world of cancer, with unexpected joy and Positude.

My hope for you is that cancer will not define who you are for the rest of your life but simply be a chapter in your epic journey.

Resources

Chapter 1 – Through The Fire

Notes
Key Statistics for Childhood Cancer

American Cancer Society – cancer.org/cancer/types/cancer-in- children/key-statistics

American Childhood Cancer Organization – acco.org

Books
The Power of Positive Thinking – Lisa R. Yanek, John Hopkins Medicine, M.P.H., 2021

Chapter 4 – Get Your Shit Together

Books
The Jester Has Lost His Jingle – David Saltzman, Jester Company, 1995

Finding online support with other parents and families:

- Facebook. Searching Facebook Groups for terms such as "childhood cancer", "pediatric oncology", or "parents of kids with cancer", for example, will return countless groups of various sizes with a host of different names. Maybe start with the larger groups, read the posts for a week, then quit the groups that aren't your jam. These groups can be great for asking nuts and bolts questions about life with childhood cancer, or for simply unloading after a particularly challenging day. Cross check and fact check any advice regarding your child's treatment or wellness with your medical team and on reputable websites like those listed below for Chapter 7.

- Momcology, from the organization's website: "Momcology has been building and maintaining responsible peer support communities for childhood cancer families since 2011. All Momcology online communities are peer moderated and conducted under support group guidelines to maintain an approachable, compassionate, and productive environment for parents seeking peer connections." momcology.org

- Stupid Cancer, a community platform for teens and young adults dealing with diagnoses, treatment, and recovery. From the organization's website: "We're here to make it all suck a little less and help you get busy living." stupidcancer.org

- The Association of Cancer Online Resources, Inc. From the organization's website: "The Association of Cancer Online Resources (ACOR) has been discontinued as a non-profit organization, but a number of its affiliated cancer mailing lists are still active." Find active and archived Listserv groups associated with a wide variety of cancers and issues. acor.org.

Finding in-person support locally:

There are many local organizations that provide professional mental health support for kids and their families, along with peer groups, activities, and some financial assistance. Ask your social worker at the hospital for more info. In the meantime, some examples of what to look for:

- Jacob's Heart – jacobsheart.org, Northern California

- Keaton's Cancer Alliance – childcancer.org, Northern California

- Childhood Cancer Foundation – ccfsocal.org, Southern California

- One Mission – onemission.org, Boston

- DC Candlelighters – dccandlelighters.org, Washington, D.C.
- Child Cancer Fund – childcancerfund.org, Northeast Florida & Southeast Georgia

Finding professionally moderated online support:

- The National Children's Cancer Society (NCCS) – thenccs.org
- Alliance for Childhood Cancer– allianceforchildhoodcancer.org
- Bear Necessities. bearnecessities.org
- The Carson Leslie Foundation – carsonlesliefoundation. org
- Children's Brain Tumor Foundation – cbtf.org
- CancerCare for Kids – cancercare.org/forkids. New York & New Jersey

Chapter 5 – Establishing Your New Normal

Notes

"Cleaning products emit hundreds of hazardous chemicals, new study finds," Environmental Working Group (EWG), News Release, September 13, 2023. ewg. org

Breathwork

Cecilia learned to calm herself for pokes by pretending to breathe like a whale—big slow breath in, hold for a couple seconds, then big slow blow out. We instructed the phlebotomist or nurse to poke on the big exhale. Worked great! Deep breathing can reduce anxiety and provide calm in any stressful situation.

- Coping Skills for Kids – copingskillsforkids.com/deep-breathing-exercises-for-kids

Mindfulness and self-hypnosis are other techniques kids can learn to calm themselves and manage the pain of pokes or other sources of anxiety.

- On YouTube, look up:

    o The Magic Glove – Hypnotic pain management for children, Dr. Leora Kuttner

    o The Body Scanner! Mindfulness for Children, The Mindfulness Teacher

    o Thought Bubbles! For Anxiety & Worry, The Mindfulness Teacher

Chemicals in Your Home

- Fundamental Hazards of Household Chemicals, Cleveland Clinic – health.clevelandclinic.org/household-cleaning-products-can-be-dangerous-to-kids-heres-how-to-use-them-safely

- DIY Cleaning Products – healthline.com/health/easy-green-diy-recipes-to-clean-all-the-things-plus-health-benefits

- Recommendations from Good Housekeeping – goodhousekeeping.com/home/cleaning/g35665355/eco-friendly-cleaning-products

Chapter 7 – Advocating For Your Child

- The Children's Oncology Group (COG). If "COG" sounds familiar, it may be because your child is being treated following a COG protocol or clinical trial, as are ninety percent of kids diagnosed each year in the U.S. Not surprisingly, there is a ton of reliable info here, including a great section on what it means to be part of a clinical trial – childrensoncologygroup.org.

- Family Handbook – childrensoncologygroup.org/ cog-family-handbook
- St. Jude, a treasure trove of information and resources for families and patients from the eminent research hospital – together.stjude.org/en-us/
- American Childhood Cancer Organization – acco.org
- The American Cancer Society, another trove of information and resources – cancer.org/cancer/survivorship/children-with-cancer/during-treatment/help-and-support.html
- Inova Health Systems, Virginia & D.C. area, has an entire website dedicated to supporting cancer patients and their families with lots of great resources – lifewithcancer.org/get-help/children-teens-and-cancer/resources-for-pediatric-oncology-patients-and-their-families/
- Alex's Lemonade Stand has a wealth of information and references – alexslemonade.org

Chapter 9 –The Hospital Party

Arts & Crafts

- Window painting kits (ask your hospital if they are allowed!)
- Coloring and sticker books and a box of markers and crayons
- Color Forms®

Toys

- Recycled butcher paper, masking tape, and markers for you and your child.

  o If they have a buddy visit, find some wall space and let them go wild with creativity!

- Invest in a few build-your-own craft kids.

   o Etsy and Amazon have fabulous and inexpensive kits of all kinds for every type of child, from flowers to science, space to animals. Check them out for inspiration. Finished art can then be used as room decor, or your child can give it to a new friend on the ward. Make sure the kits do not require strong-smelling glue as that can be difficult to tolerate on chemo.

- Nail polish kits (for both of you!)

   o Make sure that scents are okay with your roommate

- Finger paint, dot markers, paint sticks

- Stickers of all kinds and a stack of paper

- Playdough®

- Paper dolls

- Toy cars. Small (quiet) remote control cars are fun in the lobby.

- A wagon to pull around for fun!

- Bubble blowers (maybe best in lobby, outdoors, or other public spaces)

- Fold up Hot Wheels® set

Open-Ended Play

- Animal or doll sets. Look for a variety of characters your child can use for creating stories
- Wooden trains and tracks
- Felt Kids®
- Playmobil®
- Dress-up clothes. These can be as simple as a magic wand, hat, or wig, and are often fun to wear around the hospital when they feel up to moving around.

- A road or other landscape play mat
- Tea party items, blankets for forts, stuffed animals, or items for a family picnic
- Imaginext® toys
- Lego® or Duplo®
- Puppets
- Medical play set (you'd think they'd have had enough of that, but Cecilia loved reenacting procedures and interactions with her medical team, often with a stuffie or little sis as the patient—great for their mental health!)

Classic Games

- Jenga®
- Apples to Apples® card game
- Uno®
- Candyland®
- Battleship®
- Monopoly®
- Packs of kids' card games like Go Fish!

Quiet Time

- Books and audio books
- Special movies (or ones saved for hospital parties)
- Pokémon cards
- Kinetic sand
- Nintendo Switch®
- Magnet tiles
- Puzzles
- I Spy® books

- Word search puzzles or books

- Wimmel® books

- Where's Waldo® books

*Thanks to the many fellow cancer parents who contributed ideas for this list!

Music for the Hospital Party

- Music plays a big role in our family, and when songs came up on the radio in the car that spoke to us about our experience, we wrote them down. Eventually this became our playlist, Cecilia's Songs for the Journey, a mix of songs for getting fired up for a hospital party, or for when you just need to shout it out loud (see below)! Sharing a playlist on Spotify is a great way to connect with family and friends when they can't be nearby.

- Of course, before bedtime we changed the mood with music for relaxation, which you can find on countless Spotify playlists, Apple Music, Amazon Music, etc. Search playlists on your favorite streaming platform for things like "bedtime music for kids."

- As we settled in for bedtime, we always switched to a low, slow, ocean surf soundscape that remained on throughout the night, something we had always done at home since our kids were babies. Again, there are countless options for soundscapes on the music platforms. Let your child help pick one that's comforting, or maybe one that reminds them of home. Cecilia's Songs for the Journey playlist, below, can also be found on Spotify.

- *Under Pressure*, Queen with David Bowie

- *Angel*, Sarah McLachlan

- *Tubthumping*, Chumbawamba

- *Fly Away*, Lenny Kravitz
- *It's Called Courage★*, from the animated short, *Dazzle the Dinosaur*
- *Walkin' on the Sun*, Smashmouth
- *Start the Commotion*, The Wiseguys
- *I've Seen Better Days*, Barenaked Ladies
- *Lullabye*, Shawn Mullins
- *Good Riddance*, Green Day
- *Hakuna Matata*, from *The Lion King II: Simba's Pride*
- *All Star*, Smashmouth
- *Jumper*, Third Eye Blind
- *You're Still the One*, Shania Twain
- *Follow Me*, Uncle Kracker
- *We Are One*, from *Lion King 2*
- *Don't Look Back*, Boston
- *Drive*, Incubus
- *Your Life is Now*, John Mellencamp
- *All I Really Need★*, Raffi

★Not available on Spotify

Chapter 10 – Thrive, Body and Soul – Tips for You as the Caregiver

Notes

Robert Emmons, *How Gratitude Can Help You Through Hard Times, Greater Good Magazine*, May 13, 2013

Wood, A. M., et al., Gratitude and well-being: A review and theoretical integration, *Clinical Psychology Review* (2010), doi:10.1016/j.cpr.1510.03.005

The Book of Joy: Lasting Happiness in a Changing World, Tenzin Gyatso, the 14th Dalai Lama, and Archbishop Desmond Tutu, Cornerstone, 2016

Books

- *A New Earth: Awakening to Your Life's Purpose*, Eckhart Tolle, Penguin, 2005
- *Jesus Calling: Enjoying Peace in His Presence*, Sarah Young, Thomas Nelson, 2011
- *Peace is Every Step*, Thich Nhat Hanh, Random House, 1992
- *The Book of Joy: Lasting Happiness in a Changing World*, Tenzin Gyatso, the 14th Dalai Lama and Desmond Tutu, Cornerstone, 2016

Simple Self-Care for Mental Health

- Multiple clinical studies have demonstrated a high-sugar diet, or even spikes in blood sugar, can weaken our immune system, particularly concerning during chronic stress, which is itself also shown to compromise our immune system.

    o High blood sugar can impair white cell function

    o High blood sugar can trigger inflammatory responses

    o Sugar can disrupt a healthy gut biome

- Yoga

    o On YouTube, search for "Yoga with Adriene" and "Yoga Upload with Maris Aylward," two of my favorites.

    o See membership options for Peloton at onepeloton. com/membership. Note you do not need to buy any equipment from Peloton to enjoy their yoga classes.

- Earthing or Grounding
    - o For a general overview, see earthing.com
    - o The National Institutes of Health
        - The Effects of Grounding (Earthing) on Inflammation, the Immune Response, Wound Healing, and Prevention and Treatment of Chronic Inflammatory and Autoimmune Diseases, pmc.ncbi.nlm.nih.gov/articles/ PMC4378297/
        - Grounding – The Universal Anti-Inflammatory Remedy, pmc.ncbi.nlm.nih.gov/articles/ PMC10105021/
        - Earthing: Health Implications of Reconnecting the Human Body to the Earth's Surface Electrons, pmc.ncbi.nlm.nih.gov/articles/ PMC3265077/
    - o Healthline
- Grounding: Exploring Earthing Science and the Benefits Behind It, healthline.com/health/grounding
    - o WebMD
- Grounding: Techniques and Benefits, webmd.com/ balance/grounding-benefits

Chapter 11 – Thrive, Body and Soul – Tips for Your Child

Notes

Cancer and Diet 101: *How What You Eat Can Influence Cancer, Healthline*, Mary Jane Brown, PhD, RD (UK), October 7, 2018, healthline.com/nutrition/cancer-and-diet

Books

- Complementary Cancer Therapies: Combining Traditional and Alternative Approaches for the Best

Possible Outcome, Dan Labriola ND, Prima Health, 2000

Supportive Complementary Therapy

- Northwest Natural Health, Daniel Labriola ND & Lesley Morical ND, Northwest Natural Health has developed a line of supplements especially formulated for cancer patients called Safe and Sound® – nwnaturalhealth. com/suppadvanced.html

  o In our experience, NNH is a unique organization, with naturopaths collaborating side-by-side with oncologists on the cancer wards in the hospitals of the greater Seattle area. Maybe there are similar clinics near you, though we received amazing care and attention from NNH over phone and video.

  o Never provide vitamins, herbal remedies, or dietary supplements to your child without consulting the team at NNH for recommendations or without the consent of your oncology team. The protocol of chemo, radiation, etc., prescribed by your medical team is your best bet for a cure, period.

  o Complementary therapies help support the health and wellness of little bodies to better tolerate this assault and avoid secondary infections.

- Massage. Numerous studies have established the many health benefits of massage for children at any age, including simple relaxation and reduction of stress. For our warrior kids, massage can help flush lingering toxins from treatment out of muscle tissue, ease stiff joints from chemo and bed rest, and promote healthy sleep. Remember to create quiet surroundings (maybe use headphones if in-patient), start gently, and follow your child's lead for their comfort and patience. Be sure to encourage active hydration after massage to help tissues flush toxins.

- o From the National Institutes of Health: ncbi.nlm. nih.gov/pmc/articles/PMC6617372/

- o From Nationwide Children's Hospital in Columbus, Ohio: nationwidechildrens.org/ family-resources-education/700childrens/2016/02/ benefits-of-massage-therapy-for-children

- o From The Children's Hospital of Philadelphia: chop.edu/health-resources/massage

- o From Associated Bodywork & Massage Professionals: massagetherapy.com/articles/ children-and-massage

- o Video guide to simple at-home massage for children from Motion Restoration: youtube.com/playlist?list= PLpa0ewDRV5tgfqsrf9Y6ooRJZNi6lmhso

- Aromatherapy

  - o Children's Hospital of Philadelphia, *How Aromatherapy Can Help Children*, chop.edu/news/ health-tip/ how-aromatherapy-can-help-children

  - o Johns Hopkins, *Aromatherapy: Do Essential Oils Really Work?* hopkinsmedicine.org/health/ wellness-and-prevention/aromatherapy-do- essential-oils-really-work

  - o Products specifically for kids:

    - auracacia.com/kids

    - revive-eo.com/product/kids/

- Hydration, not only following massage, but especially during rounds of chemo, helps organs such as the liver and kidneys process the onslaught of toxins. Make a game of drinking an appropriate volume of water during infusion and/or immediately after, say during leucovorin rescue after methotrexate, with stickers on a sheet to mark each 20ml increment. If your child is prone to nausea and vomiting during chemo, it's even more important to replace the fluids lost as soon as they feel up to it.

- Take your child for a leisurely walk barefoot in the sand, soft dirt, or grass where it's safe to do so. This is a concept called earthing (see above) that is restorative for your body. And it's almost always therapeutic to just go outside for a walk.

- Mouth sores from chemo are especially frustrating, as the pain can be a barrier to nutrition and hydration. Here are some great tips from The MD Anderson Cancer Center: mdanderson.org/patients-family/diagnosis-treatment/emotional-physical-effects/oral-care.html

- Hair loss. This is, of course, an emotional side effect, and addressing it depends greatly on your child's age, gender, and individual temperament. Younger kids don't necessarily understand the potentially awkward social implications of baldness the way school age kids or teens might. Their "normal" is whatever world you create for them, so don't force hats and wigs on the little ones for your own comfort, for example so strangers won't stare. There's no need to make your child self-conscious about one more thing that's outside their control. For older kids and teens, don't assume they want to cover their scalp. Talk with them about how they feel, follow their lead, and support their choices with love and warmth. Some kids want to show off their shiny scalp as a badge of honor, and some fear going to school without a wig. Celebrate their individuality either way.

- The MaxLove Project, Culinary Medicine for All, maxloveproject.org
- Beads of Courage, beadsofcourage.org
- Earthing or grounding, see links above for Chapter 10

Chapter 12 – Sunshine Therapy

For Parents – addressing impacts stress, anxiety, fear and PTSD

- American Psychological Association. A great place to start. This overview provides a good orientation for taking action: apa.org/topics/children/cancer-psychological-impact
- Journal of the American Medical Association (JAMA), a thorough, though medically oriented, paper in this preeminent publication covers a study from 2010-2018 showing that cancer parents have "statistically significant increases in the probabilities of one or both parents having anxiety-related, depression-related, and any MH-related visits, respectively, compared with families of children without cancer. Such differences were greater in magnitude among mothers than fathers." – jamanetwork.com/journals/jamanetworkopen/fullarticle/2816887
- Cure Childhood Cancer, an informative article outlining how a child's cancer diagnosis can affect parents' and caregivers' relationships – curechildhoodcancer.org/blog/the-effects-of-a-childs-cancer-on-the-parents-relationship
- National Institutes of Health, article similar to the above–ncbi.nlm.nih.gov/pmc/articles/PMC8306515/
- St. Jude, a helpful guide for parents– together.stjude.org/en-us/for-families/parents/supporting-marriages.html

- Peer Reviewed Data: Systematic Review: Associations Between Family Functioning and Child Adjustment After Pediatric Cancer Diagnosis: A Meta-Analysis Marieke Van Schoors, Journal of Pediatric Psychology, Volume 42, Issue 1, January 1517

For Siblings – addressing impacts stress, anxiety, fear, and PTSD

Note that many summer camps and cancer family support centers listed above offer programs just for siblings to address their unique mental and emotional health challenges.

- University of Pennsylvania School of Nursing, an informative perspective regarding siblings' mental well-being – nursing.upenn.edu/live/news/918-seeing-cancer-through-siblings-eyes

- Sanford Health, guidelines for caring for siblings' mental well-being –news.sanfordhealth.org/childrens/the-impact-of-cancer-on-siblings/

- Canadian Cancer Society, article similar to above – cancer.ca/en/living-with-cancer/your-child-has-cancer/newly-diagnosed/how-siblings-may-react

Chapter 13 – Looking Forward

Notes

UCLA Health – uclahealth.org/news/health-benefits-gratitude

A New Earth: Awakening to Your Life's Purpose, Eckhart Tolle, Penguin, 2005

Gratitude

The American Heart Association – heart.org/en/healthy-living/healthy-lifestyle/mental-health-and-wellbeing/thankfulness-how-gratitude-can-help-your-health

The Mayo Clinic – mayoclinichealthsystem.org/hometown-health/speaking-of-health/can-expressing-gratitude-improve-health

Psychiatrist.com – psychiatrist.com/news/the-science-be-hind-the-lasting-benefits-of-gratitude

Breathing

Cyclic, or circular, breathing. For an expert video guide from Stanford University Medicine, search *How cyclic breathing can relieve stress|90 Seconds* w/ Lisa Kim on YouTube

"4-7-8 Breathing" is another simple and effective technique for re-ducing stress and anxiety – medicalnewstoday.com/articles/324417

Giving Back

For us, giving back was a great way to help process the emotional cocktail that comes with being a cancer parent, a common experience whose effects are backed by science. We had our favorite places to channel this energy as discussed earlier, but there are many ways to give back. Find the one that resonates with you!

- The American Cancer Society

    o Relay for Life. relay.org

- The Leukemia & Lymphoma Society

    o Light the Night – lightthenight.org

    o Team In Training – teamintraining.org. Note: there are ways for cancer families to be involved that don't include running a marathon!

- Make-A-Wish. wish.org

    o For your child's Wish, start with the MAW website, or ask the social worker or other staff at your hospital for help. A Wish Child needs to be recommended by their doctor or nurse practitioner. And remember, Wishes are not limited to kids with terminal diagnoses only, a common misconception.

- o Your local MAW chapter is always looking for volunteers in a wide variety of activities. You might also consider becoming a Wish Granter, which requires additional training and commitment.

- Omar's Dream Foundation enables hospitalized and medically supervised children to remotely attend school, allowing them to stay connected to their teachers and classmates. omarsdream.org

- The Deep C Podcast dives deep into childhood cancer, and is for families, caregivers, friends, and community who are supporting a child through a cancer diagnosis –thedeepcpodcast.com

- Your local cancer family support center is likely to be looking for more volunteer help, and many have annual fundraising activities you can participate in.

- St. Baldrick's Foundation, source of the original head-shaving fundraising event, now also includes other events as one of the U.S.'s biggest fundraising organizations helping support the search for cures – stbaldricks.org

- The science of positive health effects from giving back, a few examples:

  - o Columbia University Irving Medical Center – columbiadoctors.org/news/generosity-good-your-health

  - o The Cleveland Clinic – health.clevelandclinic.org/why-giving-is-good-for-your-health

  - o Rush University Medical Center – rush.edu/news/health-benefits-giving

Chapter 14 – Survivorship Begins Now

Late and Long-Term Effects

- The National Children's Cancer Society maintains a list of follow-up care programs by state – thenccs.org/long-term-clinics

- The Children's Oncology Group has an extensive index of information on possible later term effects – childrensoncologygroup.org/lateeffectsoftreatment, and guidelines for finding follow-up care for your child, https://childrensoncologygroup.org/survivorshipguidelines

Going Back to School

Getting back to school among friends, in a familiar (non-medical!) setting, and being engaged mentally and physically, are all positive goals for your child's well-being; however, navigating school protocols and getting the resources your child needs can be a difficult task. But you're now a cancer parent warrior, ready to take on the world for your kid! A few sources of help and guidelines to get you started:

- The American Cancer Society, a comprehensive overview – cancer.org/cancer/survivorship/children-with-cancer/after-treatment/returning-to-school

- The American Childhood Cancer Organization, a guide to the all-important Individualized Education Program (IEP) specifically for our kids – http://www.survivorshipguidelines.org/

- The Children's Oncology Group (COG) has extensive and comprehensive group of articles – childrensoncologygroup.org/school-support

- The Leukemia & Lymphoma Society, with Livestrong, a parent's back-to-school guide in PDF form – mskcc.org/sites/default/files/node/1228/documents/learning-livingwcancer-pdf.pdf

- The Kennedy Krieger Institute – kennedykrieger.org/stories/linking-research-classrooms-blog/supporting-childhood-cancer-survivors-school

- The National Children's Cancer Society – thenccs.org/school-parents

- CureSearch – curesearch.org/Learning-Problems-During-or-After-Treatment, and curesearch.org/Educational-Issues

Chapter 17 — Turning the Page

Notes

Robertson, I., & Cooper, C. L. (2013). Resilience [Editorial]. *Stress and Health: Journal of the International Society for the Investigation of Stress*, 29(3), 175–176.

Finding activities and camps

- Children's Oncology Camping Association has a list of over 130 camps across the U.S. and Canada – cocacamps.org

- KidsCamps, includes a list of camps in ten U.S. states as well as Canada and Ireland – kidscamps.com/special_needs/cancer_oncology.html

- Sunshine Kids, bringing activities to hospitals across the US to help kids be kids – sunshinekids.org

- Camp Okizu–Northern California, okizu.org, Family, Sibs and Bereavement Camps

- Kids & Art, programs for mental and emotional wellness through art, and a great list of camps in California – kidsandart.org

- Children's Cancer Research Fund, Minnesota, has resources and programs for families and patient wellness, including their Camp Norden – childrenscancer.org/ resources-for-families/

You can find this Resources section on this book's website, including clickable links to all the reference materials, by joining our growing community here: https://thepublishingcircle.com/ AuthorBonuses or scan this QR code: